T0344763

A Practical Guide to Vulval Disease

A Practical Guide to Vulval Disease

Diagnosis and Management

Fiona Lewis
Wexham Park Hospital
Wexham Street
Slough, UK

St John's Institute of Dermatology
Guy's & St Thomas' Hospital
London, UK

Fabrizio Bogliatto
Chivasso Civic Hospital Turin
Turin, Italy

Marc van Beurden
Netherlands Cancer Institute
Amsterdam, Netherlands

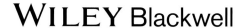

Registered Office
John Wiley & Sons Ltd, The Atrium, Southern Gate, Chichester, West Sussex, PO19 8SQ, UK

Editorial Offices
9600 Garsington Road, Oxford, OX4 2DQ, UK
The Atrium, Southern Gate, Chichester, West Sussex, PO19 8SQ, UK.
111 River Street, Hoboken, NJ 07030-5774, USA

For details of our global editorial offices, for customer services and for information about how to apply for permission to reuse the copyright material in this book please see our website at www.wiley.com/wiley-blackwell.

Library of Congress Cataloging-in-Publication Data

Names: Lewis, Fiona, 1963– author. | Bogliatto, Fabrizio, author. | Beurden, Marc van, author.
Title: Practical guide to vulval disease : diagnosis and management / Fiona Lewis, Fabrizio Bogliatto, Marc van Beurden.
Description: Chichester, West Sussex ; Hoboken, NJ : John Wiley & Sons, Inc., 2017. | Includes bibliographical references and index.
Identifiers: LCCN 2016040293 (print) | LCCN 2016040776 (ebook) | ISBN 9781119146056 (cloth) | ISBN 9781119146063 (pdf) | ISBN 9781119146070 (epub)
Subjects: | MESH: Vulvar Diseases | Vulva–pathology
Classification: LCC RG261 (print) | LCC RG261 (ebook) | NLM WP 200 | DDC 618.1/6–dc23
LC record available at https://lccn.loc.gov/2016040293

A catalogue record for this book is available from the British Library.

Cover image: *Pazhyna/Gettyimages*

Set in 10/12pt Warnock by SPi Global, Pondicherry, India
Printed and bound in Singapore by Markono Print Media Pte Ltd

10 9 8 7 6 5 4 3 2 1

Contents

Acknowledgements

We would like to thank all those who have helped us with the preparation of this book – particularly our trainees who inspired us to write it and our colleagues for their encouragement.

Our thanks to Dr Catherine Stefanato for supplying the immunofluorescence figures, Figures 16.3 and 16.4, and to Dr Eduardo Calonje, Marie-Laure Jullie and Kristina Semkova for help with the photography of histology slides. We are also indebted to Dr Joris Hage for providing the clinical photographs in Figures 20.5a and 21.2.

We are grateful to our patients who have allowed us to use their clinical photographs and to our medical photography colleagues for their patience, advice and technical skills.

1

The Normal Vulva

The vulva is a complex organ, due to its embryologic derivation from the three germ layers belonging to the embryonic disc:

- ectoderm (squamous epithelium);
- mesoderm (connective epithelium);
- endoderm (vulval vestibule).

This embryological derivation is responsible for the different variants in morphology that occur during the development of the vulva.

A correct and thorough knowledge of the 'normal' vulva is vital for several reasons. Firstly, it is important in order to recognize some of the normal anatomical variants in order to differentiate them from pathological features. This will prevent unnecessary excision and treatment of normal areas. Secondly, it leads to a more specific and logical approach in treating vulval disorders. In some conditions, the normal anatomy of the vulva is altered and this can give diagnostic clues. It is important to note that the 'normal' vulva modifies itself during a woman's lifetime, depending on age, obstetrical and gynaecological history.

Normal Vulval Anatomy

The vulva may be considered as the combination of the mucosal, cutaneous, muscular and connective tissue structures that compose the lower part of the female genital tract. The peculiarity of this localization means that the vulva is in close association with urological structures (urethra and bladder), gynaecological structures (vagina), and intestinal structures (rectum and anus).

The borders of the vulva are: mons pubis anteriorly, perineal body posteriorly, genital crural folds laterally and hymen medially (Figure 1.1). In this triangular-shaped region, with naked-eye examination, five distinct structures clearly appear: the labia majora, the clitoris, the vestibule, the labia minora and the hymen (Figure 1.2 a, b).

There is usually a limited description of the internal structures of the vulva in gynaecological and dermatological textbooks. These structures reach the plane of the perineal fascia (or urogenital membrane) under the skin. A knowledge of the anatomy of these structures and planes then encompasses the clitoral body, the minor vestibular bulbs and glands, the urethral opening and the paraurethral glands, which are all part of the vulva. A good understanding of the anatomy, together with its embryological development, allows a comprehensive approach to vulval morphology and correct surgical dissection if required.

A Practical Guide to Vulval Disease: Diagnosis and Management, First Edition. Fiona Lewis, Fabrizio Bogliatto and Marc van Beurden.

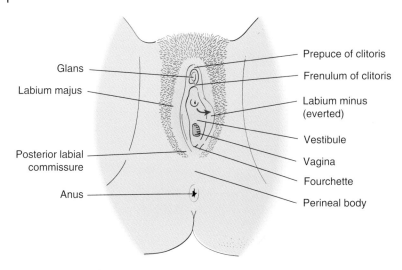

Figure 1.1 The vulva.

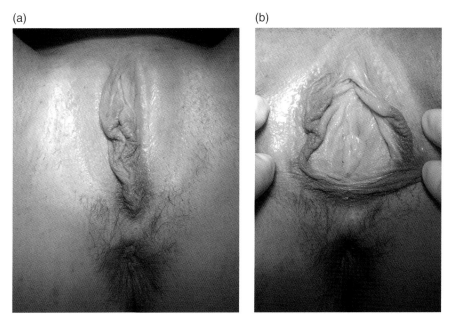

Figure 1.2 Normal vulva (a) – outer and (b) – inner vulva.

The **labia majora** are two cutaneous folds, even and symmetrical, arising from the lateral portions of the mons pubis and extending to the posterior triangle of the perineum. Laterally they terminate on the genito-crural fold, and medially continue to the external aspects of the labia minora, forming the interlabial sulci. On the outer surface, they are covered by hair-bearing skin. The hair follicles are lost on the inner surface but many sebaceous glands remain.

The **labia minora** are two thin structures that are connected anteriorly to form the clitoral hood and, below the clitoral body, form the frenulum. Posteriorly the labia minora unite to define the fourchette The epithelium starting from the internal side of the fourchette to the hymen is called the navicular fossa. The labia minora do not have hair follicles but they are covered by numerous sebaceous glands and sweat glands.

The *clitoris* develops from an outgrowth in the embryo called the genital tubercle. It contains trabeculated erectile tissue, similar to the male penis, and is composed of the body (the shaft and the glans) and the crura. The glans is covered by the clitoral hood, formed by the fusion of the anterior portions of the labia minora. The body of the clitoris continues in each crus (singular form of 'crura'), attached to the corresponding ischial ramus, beneath the descending pubic rami. Hence only about 30% of the clitoris is visible (Figure 1.3).

The *vestibule* is the space between the hymenal ring and the internal aspect of labia minora. Its boundaries are the clitoris anteriorly, the fourchette posteriorly and the 'Hart's line' laterally, which runs down the internal side of the labia minora. It represents the junction between the mucosal epithelium and the keratinized skin of the vestibule (Figure 1.4). Some authors define the lateral extension of the vestibule as the free edge of labia minora, therefore including the two types of epithelium (mucosa and skin).

Several structures open into the vestibule. The urethral opening is clearly seen with the paraurethral Skene's glands laterally. The ducts of the Bartholin's glands and the lesser vestibular glands open into the lower third of the vaginal introitus.

The bulb of the vestibule is located deeply and, as aggregations of erectile tissue, this may be considered as an internal part of the clitoris.

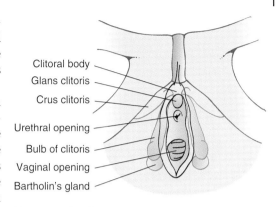

Figure 1.3 The clitoris.

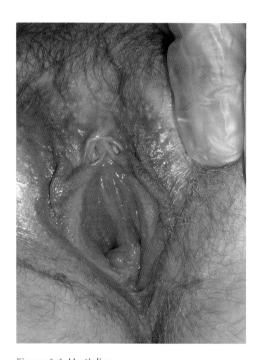

Figure 1.4 Hart's line.

The *hymen* is an elastic ring-shaped structure, covered by mucosal epithelium that separates the vagina from the vulval vestibule. After the first penetrative sexual intercourse it can be torn apart, leaving one or more scars on its surface. Very rarely the hymen may be septate or cribriform.

The *mons pubis* lies in front of and above the upper part of the symphysis pubis. A thick cushion of subcutaneous fat is covered by hair-bearing keratinized epithelium.

The vulva obtains its blood supply from the internal pudendal artery and drains via the external pudendal vein. The nerve supply is from branches of the perineal nerve but the clitoris is supplied by the dorsal nerve of the clitoris, a branch of the pudendal nerve. Lymphatic drainage is to the inguinal and internal iliac nodes.

Normal Vulval and Vaginal Flora

The vagina is colonized by several strains of bacteria. At puberty, lactobacilli increase and the glycogen metabolized by them produces lactic acid, giving a normal vaginal acidic pH of 4.5 or less. A change in the normal discharge can occur if levels of *Candida albicans* or *Streptococcus agalactiae* (beta haemolytic streptococcus) increase but this does not necessarily require any treatment.

Further Reading

Andrikopoulou, M., Michala, L. and Creighton, S. M. (2013) The normal vulva in medical textbooks. *Journal of Obstetrics and Gynaecology* **33**, 648–650.

Lloyd, J., Crouch, N. S., Minto, C. L. *et al.* (2005) Female genital appearance: 'normality' unfolds. *British Journal of Obstetrics and Gynaecology* **112**, 643–646.

Neill, S. M. and Lewis, F. M. (2009) Basics of vulval embryology, anatomy and physiology, in *Ridley's The Vulva*, 3rd edn (eds S. M. Neill and F. M. Lewis). Wiley-Blackwell, London, pp. 13–33.

Normal Anatomical Variants

The shape and morphology of the vulva depend on the appearance of all the structures involved. The differences in the developmental process and integration into the whole of each structure render the vulva a unique organ. For this reason it is usual to find some variants; that should be considered normal. However, these can cause great worry to a woman when she first looks at her vulva. In addition, the explosion in cosmetic surgery for the external genitalia in recent years in order to reach a 'perfect vulva' has greatly increased the focus of attention on vulval appearance. As a consequence, aesthetic vulval surgery is performed, modifying structures that are normal, without any pathological reason.

Common normal vulval variants are considered here.

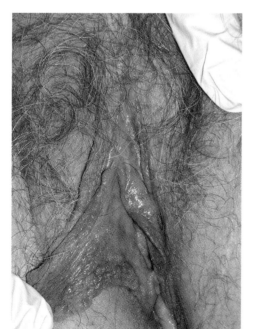

Figure 1.5 Bifid labium minus.

- *Agenesis of the labia minora.* This is a normal finding in women but should not be confused with labial adhesion. The latter condition is an acquired disease, more frequent in girls under 2 years due to several predisposing factors such as oestrogen deprivation, inadequate personal care, local irritants, infections or previous trauma. This situation may mimic labial reabsorption in lichen sclerosus but generally resolves spontaneously.
- *Asymmetry of the labia minora.* There is great variability in the size and shape of the labia minora. In one study, the length and width of the labia minora were examined in 50 women aged from 18 to 50. The length varied from 20 to 100 mm and the width from 7 to 50 mm. Sometimes a duplication of the labia minora may occur, without any pathological consequence (Figure 1.5). The edge of the labia minora may become rugose and the rim is often pigmented.

- **Sebaceous glands.** The vulva is rich in sebaceous glands (Fordyce spots) that can appear as little yellow spots spread on the vestibule and labia minora (Figure 1.6). In some cases, hypertrophic and inflamed sebaceous glands may upset the normal surface anatomy of the labia. This condition is known as Fox–Fordyce disease.
- **Vestibular papillomatosis.** Often misdiagnosed and treated as HPV condylomata, this condition is characterized by papillary growths of the vestibular mucosa located within Hart's line. On naked eye examination, they are finger-like projections and each has a solitary base (Figure 1.7).
- **Vestibular erythema.** Located in the vestibule at the opening of the Bartholin glands, this physiological erythema is found, in observational studies, in more than 40% of asymptomatic women. Previously associated with localized provoked vestibular pain, it is now to be considered a normal variant.
- **Paraurethral cysts and vestibular cysts.** Cysts of Skene's glands or paraurethral cysts are a normal finding and are often asymptomatic. In case of excessive growth, surgical excision may be indicated. These conditions may mimic vulval cancer but the regular shape, the softness on palpation and the normal lining should lead to a correct diagnosis.
- **Membranous fourchette (membrane like).** Occasionally, where the posterior labia minora join (fourchette) this can be thinned and looks like a thin band of mucous membrane. This is a normal finding, usually causing no problems during intercourse or gynaecological examination. In some cases, however, particularly after the menopause or in some oestrogen-depleted states with atrophy, the membranous fourchette may become symptomatic, especially during intercourse, requiring topical oestrogens or surgical therapy.
- **Clitoral hood.** The shape and the size of the clitoris and clitoral hood have a great variability. Sometimes the hood is covered by transitional epithelium, rendering this structure more sensitive (it is estimated to have more than 8000 sensory nerve endings).
- **Hair distribution.** The distribution of pubic hair has a wide spectrum, depending on race and age. It varies in colour and in distribution, tending to become thinner in older age. In young women, pubic hair removal may cause irritation, mimicking candida infection, or cause folliculitis. If hair is absent at any age, the differential diagnosis is alopecia and needs further investigation.
- **Colour of the vulva.** The genital area is characterized by an increased number of melanocytes in comparison to other areas of the body. A darker

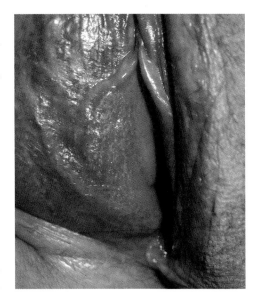

Figure 1.6 Fordyce spots.

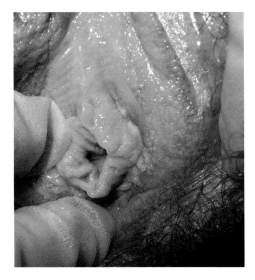

Figure 1.7 Vestibular papillomatosis.

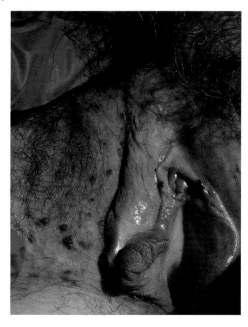

Figure 1.8 Angiokeratomata.

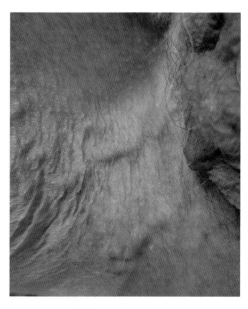

Figure 1.9 Vulval varicosities.

skin of the vulva, particularly localized in the labia minora and clitoral hood, is normal.

- **Angiokeratomas.** These are very common small vascular papules usually seen on the labia majora (Figure 1.8). They are asymptomatic and should not be diagnosed and managed as genital warts or cancer. No biopsy is required. They may disappear with gentle digital pressure.
- **Vulval varicosities.** Varicosities of the labial veins may be unilateral or bilateral and are seen on the outer labia majora (Figure 1.9). They may appear in pregnancy.

Normal Changes Over the Lifetime

Childhood

In the infant, the labia minora are poorly developed and the vestibule is more exposed. No hair is seen. At puberty, the labia majora and mons pubis become more prominent due to the deposition of fat. Pubic hair growth develops the adult pattern between the ages of 12 and 17.

Pregnancy

Increased progesterone predisposes to venous distension and hence the development of vulval varicosities. Increased pigmentation is common, especially in darker skin types. Immune dysregulation may lead to an increased incidence of infection such as candidiasis.

Menopause

The density of hair growth is reduced and the labia majora become less prominent due to a reduction in subcutaneous fat. The loss of oestrogen leads to a thinning of the epithelium with consequent dryness and increased fragility. Associated urinary incontinence can cause significant problems with irritancy.

Further Reading

Dhawan AK, Pandhi, D., Goyal, S. and Bisherwal, K. (2014) Angiokeratoma of vulva mimicking genital warts. *Journal of Obstetrics and Gynaecology of India* **64** (suppl 1), 148–149.

Farage, M. and Maibach, H. (2006) Lifetime changes in the vulva and vagina. *Archives of Gynecology and Obstetrics* **273**, 195–202.

Moyal-Barracco, M., Leibowitch, M. and Orth, G. (1990) Vestibular papillae of the vulva: lack of evidence for human papilloma virus aetiology. *Archives of Dermatology* **126**, 1594–1598.

Van Beurden, M., van der Vange, N., de Craen, A. J. *et al.* (1997) Normal findings in vulvar examination and vulvoscopy. *British Journal of Obstetrics and Gynaecology* **104**(3), 320–324.

2

Taking a History and Examination

Taking a History

Taking a good history is fundamental in the diagnosis and management of any patient presenting with vulval symptoms. This step is the keystone for the clinical diagnosis and for establishing the doctor–patient relationship.

It is important to recognize that there are several factors that can make the history difficult to obtain in full. Older patients are reluctant to give intimate information. The presence of nonspecific symptoms such as itching, burning and pain can lead to confusion of the clinical picture and the short time for the consultation is often inadequate to evaluate the emotional aspects of the problem for a complete psychosexual assessment. Some of these issues may only become apparent during further follow-up consultations.

First of all, it is important to use the right setting, choosing a quiet and discrete ambient area without disturbance. In establishing an initial rapport with the patient, the healthcare professional should be approachable with a friendly manner. After introducing yourself, it is important to explain the reason for the interview, seeking consent for taking notes, and demonstrating respect for, and interest in, the patient's problem.

Ensure that there is correct identification of the patient with the date and place of birth. Open questions are useful initially to identify the patient's major symptoms, focusing later on the specific reasons for attending for consultation. Show that you are listening, make eye contact with the patient, tailor the questions to the information being given, and reflect back what the patient is saying, using concise and easily understood language. The patient is often unfamiliar with the different parts of the vulva and they frequently use the term 'vagina' to describe the external genitalia. Try to discuss the anatomy of the vulva and the localization of the disease in a simple manner and clarify statements and jargon used by the patient.

To obtain all the clinical information it is suitable to start with an enquiry about the general medical history, followed by the gynaecological and dermatological history and, at the end, to explore a specific history about the vulval problem.

General Medical History

- General medical condition and past medical history.
- Family history of disease.
- History of allergic disease such as asthma or hay fever.
- History of systemic, metabolic, autoimmune diseases. Diabetes, especially if poorly controlled, should deserve special attention in the investigation of some common vulval symptoms such as pruritus.

A Practical Guide to Vulval Disease: Diagnosis and Management, First Edition. Fiona Lewis, Fabrizio Bogliatto and Marc van Beurden.
© 2017 John Wiley & Sons Ltd. Published 2017 by John Wiley & Sons Ltd.

- It is useful to check for any medical prescriptions, for drugs taken orally or used topically in the previous 6 months. This should also include self-administered preparations and those bought over the counter.
- Smoking history – this is very important as smoking is a significant risk factor in those with vulval intraepithelial neoplasia or hidradenitis suppurativa.
- Travel history – this may be relevant to some rare infections.
- A record of body mass index (BMI) is of particular importance because obesity affects vulval physiology with its unfavourable effect of increased friction on the skin potentially leading to maceration. This can then predispose to infections such as candidiasis. Hygiene practices may also be ineffective if the patient cannot reach the area adequately.

Gynaecological History

- Menstrual history – record the age of the first menses and, if relevant, the menopause
- Results of cervical cytology tests and any abnormalities or treatment required.
- Pregnancy – the number of pregnancies (including terminations and miscarriages) and mode of delivery. Any lacerations or problems after the delivery should be noted.
- Habits regarding hygiene and clothing.
- Mode of contraception should be noted, if relevant.
- Enquire about any previous sexually transmitted diseases or recurring infections.
- Presence of genital or anal prolapse, or urinary incontinence with daily use of pads should be checked.
- Any surgical procedures on the lower genital tract, radiotherapy or chemotherapy should be recorded.

Dermatological History

- Previous skin disease, especially eczema or psoriasis, treatment used and the response.
- Contact allergy. Enquire about previous patch testing and the results.
- Family history of skin disease.

Vulval History

This is made up of two specific steps focused on the *symptom* itself and then on *detailed information* regarding that symptom including time of onset; correlation to specific events (triggering and alleviating factors), hygiene or clothing habits, sporting activity and the use of topical preparations may be helpful in leading to the diagnosis.

Investigation of vulval symptoms includes:

- Definition of symptoms: pain, burning, itching, soreness.
- Evolution of the condition: is it acute or chronic? Is there exacerbation during the day or night? Did it start in one area and then spread or is it localized?
- Associated events – vaginal discharge, urinary infection, similar symptoms elsewhere. Information on the patient's washing and cleaning habits used in the last 3 months is very useful as certain foams, soaps, or creams may cause a chronic irritant reaction. In addition, many patients will wash more frequently when they have vulval symptoms and excessive cleansing can modify the skin hydrolipid biofilm with consequent local irritation. Clothing habits (wearing tight pants, coloured and synthetic clothes and pads), with increased perspiration in the area, can also add to local irritation.

- Associated cutaneous or mucosal lesions
- Response to treatment (use/abuse of topical preparations)
- Impact on lifestyle

In the investigation of vulval pain, the main points to cover can easily be remembered using the mnemonic 'SOCRATES':

S – site (localized, generalized);
O – onset (after vaginal infection, or specific event);
C – character (continuous, intermittent);
R – radiation (back, bladder, rectus);
A – associations;
T – timing;
E – exacerbating and relieving factors;
S – severity.

When you have completed the history taking, explain to the patient that, to reach a diagnosis, it is important to proceed to a good clinical examination of the vulva, using vulvoscopy if required. A chaperone should always be present and there are clear guidelines relating to the use of chaperones. Explain to the patient that a biopsy may be needed and full informed consent should be taken and documented. Similarly, inform the patient about the necessity to take a clinical picture of the vulva for their medical records.

Examination of the Vulva

Any patient with a vulval complaint should be evaluated by someone who is familiar with the specific problems that can occur at this site. This includes the dermatological, infective, psychosexual and gynaecological disorders that affect the genital tract. The use of the colposcope and the application of acetic acid, toluidine blue or both adds little or nothing to naked-eye examination of the vulva. The vulva, unlike the cervix and anus, is composed of skin and keratinized epithelium and there is no transformation zone. Therefore, application of acetic acid on the cutaneous and mucous epithelium of vulva, as it is a nontransitional epithelium, is not only unhelpful but can be misleading. Other colour tests, such as toluidine blue or Lugol's iodine, do not have any substantial benefit. Furthermore, toluidine blue (Collins test) gives a high percentage of false positive results on inflammatory lesions and ulcers and false negative results, especially on high-grade vulval intraepithelial neoplastic lesions.

The term vulvoscopy is appropriate and useful because it is easy to comprehend. However, vulvoscopy should be defined as a composite diagnostic tool that includes careful naked-eye and low-power magnified examination carried out by those with interdisciplinary skills. It should be considered as the macroscopic observation of the vulval and perineal skin and not as the colposcopic inspection of the vulva after application of acetic acid. Occasionally the colposcope is useful as a lens, especially to evaluate flexural sites. A good lamp with central magnification is perfectly adequate for examination of the vulva and is used by most dermatologists (Figure 2.1).

Examination of the vulva should follow a sequential method for every patient, in order to reach a final and precise diagnosis. Firstly, the vulva is inspected and then it is possible to proceed to palpation, explaining to the patient all the actions to be performed. Examination should be conducted without causing pain or discomfort and this can be achieved by asking the patient if she has any pain and by palpating gently to start with. Remember to look at the patient's face

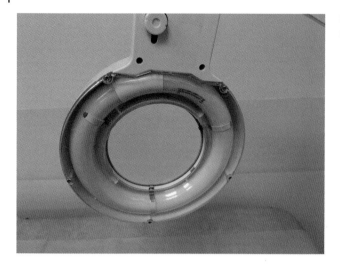

Figure 2.1 A lamp with good light and magnification is vital.

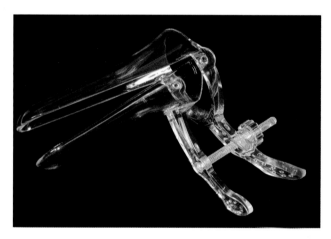

Figure 2.2 Plastic speculum.

when you are feeling for tenderness. This is especially important in those patients presenting with vulval pain, which may be provoked by touch.

Inspection starts at the vestibule by opening widely the labia minora. Check the hymen, the urethral meatus and the inner surfaces of the labia minora. Then check the free edge and the external surfaces of the labia minora together with the clitoral hood and the fourchette, moving to the inter-labial sulci and then the inner aspects of the labia majora. Complete the examination with the inspection of the hair-bearing surfaces of the labia majora, mons pubis, genito-crural folds and finally the perineum. Extend the inspection to the anal and perianal zones and palpate the inguinal regions too if necessary.

In many cases, such as those presenting with erosive disease or possible vulval intraepithelial neoplasia, it is vital to examine the vagina to check for disease at this site. The plastic speculum (Figure 2.2) is very helpful as this will provide a good view of the vaginal mucosa. For any dermatosis, a full skin examination can give important diagnostic clues. Examination of other mucous membranes, for example the mouth and lacrimal ducts is also important. In some situations, further specialist examination may be required such as proctoscopy or conjunctival examination and the patient should be referred to the appropriate specialist.

This examination should then detect any abnormality and details must be documented (see Chapter 8):

- colour change – red or white areas, hypo- or hyper- pigmented areas;
- surface – papules or plaques, nodules, vesicles or bullae;
- loss of tissue and any loss of normal anatomy;
- erosions or ulcers.

When a lesion is detected, it is necessary to evaluate the thickness, the infiltration and the mobility.

The features can be documented by a simple clinical drawing but clinical photographs are very useful in the medical report because the most accurate written description is often subjective and can vary, even if performed by the same physician. In addition, photographs allow the monitoring of any change in a lesion with time, the efficacy of therapy, and the development of new lesions They also represent a vital tool for a discussion with clinical colleagues and pathologists.

Further Reading

Micheletti, L., Bogliatto, F. and Lynch, P, J. (2008) Vulvoscopy. Review of diagnostic approach requiring clarification. *Journal of Reproductive Medicine* **53**, 179–182.

Neill, S. M. and Lewis, F. M. (2009) Principles of examination, investigation and treatment, in *Ridley's The Vulva*, 3rd edn (eds S. M. Neill and F. M. Lewis). Wiley-Blackwell, London, pp. 34–37.

Royal College of Obstetricians and Gynaecologists (1997) *Intimate Examinations: A Report of a Working Party*, Royal College of Obstetricians and Gynaecologists, London

Van Beurden, M., van der Vange, N., de Craen, A. J. *et al.* (1997) Normal findings in vulvar examination and vulvoscopy. *British Journal of Obstetrics and Gynaecology* **104**(3), 320–324.

3

How to Take a Vulval Biopsy and the Importance of Clinico-Pathological Correlation

A vulval biopsy may be performed for several reasons: to confirm the clinical diagnosis, to differentiate between clinical diagnoses when it is not possible to be certain on the basis of clinical features alone, and to aid in making a clear diagnosis where the clinical signs are atypical. A vulval biopsy should not be performed in isolation without considering the clinical signs and symptoms. Taking a biopsy and sending it to a pathologist for a diagnosis without any clinical information is dangerous as the wrong conclusions can easily be drawn. The biopsy should be accompanied by an accurate description of the clinical examination (supplied by pictures) and the clinical diagnostic hypothesis. This information is essential for the pathologist to interpret the histopathological features of vulval lesions correctly.

Many vulval problems are dermatological diseases, so ideally an expert dermatopathologist should report the histology, or at least be available to discuss difficult cases. The environment of the vulva, with heat and moisture, can modify some histological features, making it more difficult to make a diagnosis. The application of topical treatment before the biopsy can alter the histopathological signs. A multidisciplinary approach involving pathologists, gynaecologists and dermatologists is fundamental to overcome possible misunderstanding and to allow for clinico-pathological correlation.

Biopsy can be incisional or excisional. In the first case, the biopsy has a specific diagnostic purpose; in the second case, it can also have a therapeutic role. The site of a biopsy must be chosen carefully. For example, it is unhelpful to biopsy the base of an ulcer or erosion because the most useful diagnostic histological features are likely to be found at the edge of the lesion. Specific issues relating to biopsy site are detailed in subsequent chapters.

Before taking the biopsy, check that the patient does not have any coagulopathy or allergy to local anaesthetic. It is important to explain the procedure and to obtain informed consent.

A sterile technique is used and the first step is adequate disinfection of the skin or mucosa to prevent infection (Figure 3.1). Iodine is often used but a colourless and foam free antiseptic such as chlorhexidine is useful to maintain a clear vision of the lesion. If necessary, the hair should be removed.

The use of an injectable local anaesthetic such as 1–2% lidocaine, is always required. Topical local anaesthetic cream may be used for small biopsies in the vestibule and is sometimes used to reduce the pain of injecting the local anaesthetic at other vulval sites. However, it is again vital that the pathologist knows the usual practice of the clinician, as pathological artefacts induced by EMLA® (prilocaine/lidocaine mixture) can lead to major diagnostic pitfalls. Infiltration (2–5 ml) is performed with subepidermal injection using a thin 30-gauge needle (Figure 3.2).

A Practical Guide to Vulval Disease: Diagnosis and Management, First Edition. Fiona Lewis, Fabrizio Bogliatto and Marc van Beurden.
© 2017 John Wiley & Sons Ltd. Published 2017 by John Wiley & Sons Ltd.

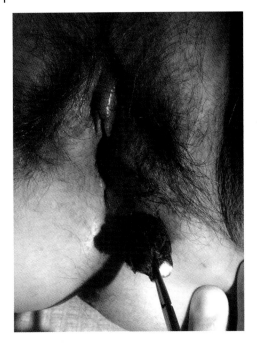

Figure 3.1 The area to be biopsied is cleaned with antiseptic.

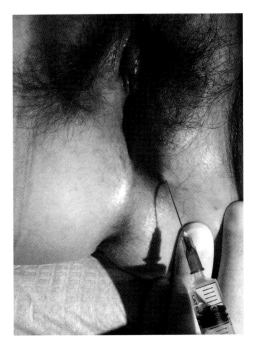

Figure 3.2 Local anaesthetic is infiltrated.

Incisional Biopsy

The cold-knife or Keye's punch (Figure 3.3) are the most suitable tools for a correct vulval incisional biopsy. Shave biopsies are not adequate for diagnosis, particularly for inflammatory dermatoses. In general, ***punch biopsies*** are easy to perform, can be done in an outpatient setting and are suitable for the diagnosis of most dermatoses. The minimum size should be 4 mm. The skin is slightly stretched and the punch biopsy inserted (Figure 3.4) and rotated to provide a small core of tissue (Figure 3.5) It is important not to crush the sample as it is removed.

The biopsy specimen must be representative of the whole lesion: it should not be too small and should have an adequate depth. The optimal depth is approximately 5 mm in normal skin conditions but in cases of hyperkeratosis the depth is related to adjacent normal skin in order to avoid the sample being too superficial. It should always include dermal papillae in order to permit an accurate measurement of the depth of the lesion, which is particularly useful in the diagnosis of intraepithelial neoplastic lesions and extramammary Paget's disease.

Cold-knife biopsy allows shaping of the depth and width of the specimen. This is optimal when including an area of healthy tissue around the lesion that could be needed for histological comparison of lesional and nonlesional tissue (Figures 3.6, 3.7 and 3.8). This is the most appropriate method for obtaining a specimen that needs direct immunofluorescence examination, as the elliptical biopsy can be halved horizontally with the lesional skin being sent for histological examination and the nonlesional tissue for immuno-fluorescence studies.

Haemostasis can be achieved with the apposition of the edges of the biopsy site and then sutured with absorbable sutures of vicryl 3-0 or 5-0 (Figures 3.9 and 3.10).

These biopsies heal within 5–7 days and the sutures generally absorb in 10 days. Aftercare is important if the biopsy is in a site where faecal contamination may be an issue. Gentle cleaning twice daily is helpful, using 1% chlorhexidine foam or detergent.

The cervical biopsy forceps, which are very useful on the cervical and vaginal mucosa, must not be used on the vulva as they produce samples that are unsuitable

Figure 3.3 Punch biopsy.

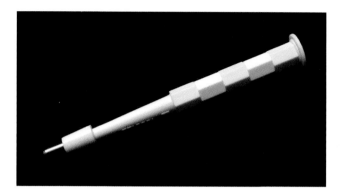

Figure 3.4 The punch biopsy is inserted and rotated.

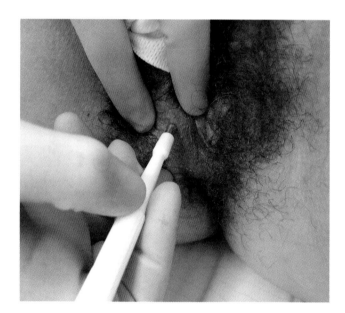

Figure 3.5 A core of tissue is obtained and cut off at the base.

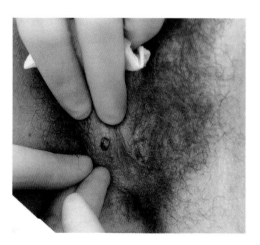

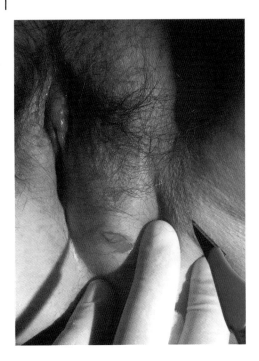

Figure 3.6 Cold knife biopsy – ellipse is cut.

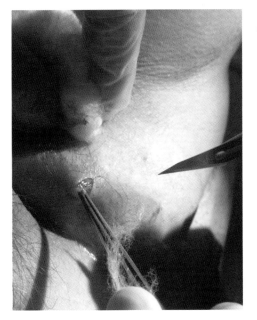

Figure 3.7 Cold knife biopsy – the ellipse is then excised to a depth of at least 5 mm.

for accurate histological analysis. Loop or needle electrode and CO_2 laser are valid alternative methods, comparable to cold knife, which allow for modulation in depth and width of the biopsy sample but can cause heat artefacts, which can compromise histological interpretation. They may be useful for haemostasis or removing small nodular exophytic benign lesions.

Figure 3.8 The surgical wound that results.

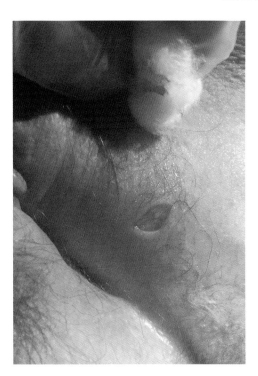

Figure 3.9 Haemostasis is achieved by suturing.

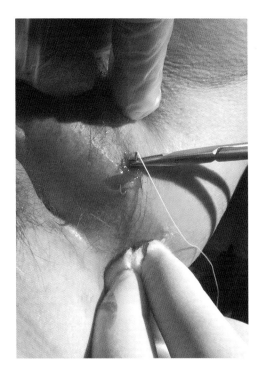

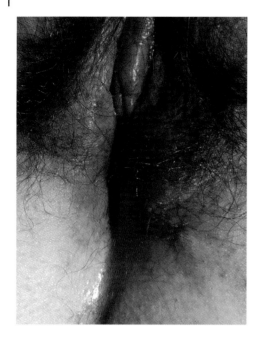

Figure 3.10 The final appearance.

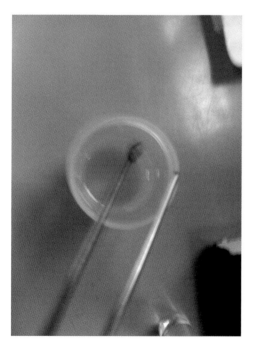

Figure 3.11 The tissue is then immediately put into fixative.

Fixation of the Biopsy

The biopsy specimen, independently of the technique, should be placed immediately in a fixative medium (Figure 3.11) in order to avoid deterioration, making analysis impossible. Formalin 10% or alcohol are generally used, avoiding Bouin's fixative, which can invalidate immunohistochemical reactions. The time of fixation is variable: small samples of 3–4 mm may need only 1–2 h, but wide excisions require 12–14 h. Samples for immunofluorescence should be placed in Michel's medium where they are stable for up to 28 days.

Crushed specimens can cause problems with the laboratory histological cut–up procedure, producing oblique or flat microtome sections. This can result in absence of the dermis, making it impossible to evaluate the depth of the lesion necessary in the diagnosis of malignancy, such as invasive or intra-epithelial neoplasia, or to assess involvement of appendageal structures.

Orientation of the specimen with the use of a suture or coloured mark, together with a picture of the lesion, facilitates correct evaluation by the pathologist.

The request form, sent with the sample, is important. The biographical data of the patient must correspond with those that identify the sample. The clinical history, a description of the lesion and the clinical diagnosis or differential diagnosis should be documented.

Before processing, the pathologist will examine the sample, giving a macroscopic description of the lesion. Small samples (3-4 mm), laid down on a support of embedding synthetic material to prevent deformation, should be entirely processed. Larger biopsies should be cut in several parts, taking care to guide the cut on the vertical axis. The histological sections are then stained with haematoxylin and eosin. Further tests including immuno-staining or *in situ* hybridization or PCR for infective agents may be needed on the basis of the H&E histological features.

Further Reading

Goldstein, G. P. and Goldstein, A. (2009) Punch biopsy for the evaluation of vulvar dermatoses. *Journal of Sexual Medicine* **6**, 1214–1217.

Irvin, W. and Taylor, P. (2004) Biopsy of lesions of the female genital tract in the ambulatory setting. *Journal of Long-Term Effects of Medical Implants* **14**, 185–199.

Lewis, F.M., Agarwal, A., Neill, S. M. *et al.* (2013) The spectrum of histopathologic patterns secondary to the topical application of EMLA® on vulvar epithelium: clinic-pathologic correlation in 3 cases. *Journal of Cutaneous Pathology* **40**, 708–713.

Lynch, P. J. and Edwards, L. (1994) *Genital Dermatology*, Churchill Livingstone, New York, NY, pp. 7–9.

4

Basic Histology of the Vulva

The vulva has both keratinized and nonkeratinized (mucosal) epithelium. On the labia majora, mons pubis and perineal region, the epithelium is keratinized and is similar to skin at other body sites. The keratinocytes move upwards through the epidermis and are eventually shed. Four distinct layers can be seen in the epithelium – from bottom to top, basal layer, stratum spinosum, stratum granulosum and, most superficially, the stratum corneum. Skin appendages at these sites include hair follicles, eccrine glands (producing odourless and colourless sweat), apocrine glands (producing a milk-like odourless secretion, which, due to bacterial action, can release pheromones) and sebaceous glands (Figure 4.1). These appendageal structures vary in their localization. The skin covering the outer surfaces of the labia majora is rich in hair follicles, sebaceous glands, eccrine and apocrine glands. The inner surface has no hair follicles or apocrine glands but several sebaceous glands and some eccrine glands (this is the only region apart from the nipples where sebaceous glands are found without hair). The absence of hair allows the sebaceous glands to be visible to the naked eye and present clinically as slight yellow bumps, called Fordyce spots (see Chapter 1).

The epithelium that covers the hymen, vestibule and inner surfaces of the labia minora is a nonkeratinized mucosal type. Adnexal structures are absent but sebaceous glands are common on the labia minora. Sometimes pigmentation, due to an increase in the number of melanocytes with a high quantity of melanin, occurs on the outer surfaces of the labia minora and on the clitoral hood. The vestibular mucosa is rich in glycogen and it is important not to confuse this with koilicytosis seen with human papilloma infection.

Three other types of cells are present in the epithelium.

- Langerhans cells are derived from the bone marrow and are very important as antigen-presenting cells, playing a part in contact dermatitis and immune surveillance.
- Merkel cells have an irregular distribution and have a close relationship with afferent nerve fibres. Their precise role is not known.
- Melanocytes are derived from the neural crest and produce melanin pigments. They migrate to the external genital region during foetal life and are seen in vulval epithelium in varying numbers. They are increased in patients with darker skin and also increase during pregnancy when hormonal changes stimulate increased melanogenesis.

In approaching the diagnosis of a patient with a vulval disorder it is necessary for the clinician to know the terms that are used to describe the cell types and histopathological features of the disease, in order to achieve clear communication with the pathologist.

Tables 4.1 and 4.2 contain glossaries of the principal terms used in the pathological description, and some of the more common special stains used to confirm a diagnosis.

A Practical Guide to Vulval Disease: Diagnosis and Management, First Edition. Fiona Lewis, Fabrizio Bogliatto and Marc van Beurden.
© 2017 John Wiley & Sons Ltd. Published 2017 by John Wiley & Sons Ltd.

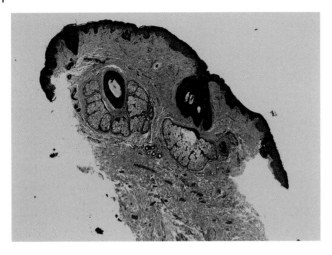

Figure 4.1 Histopathological features of the normal vulva.

Table 4.1 Glossary of cell types and structures.

			Commonly seen in
Basement membrane	Junction between epidermis and dermis	Can be visualized with PAS stain	
Epidermal giant cells	Multinucleate keratinocytes		Herpes virus infection
Epithelioid cells	They look similar to keratinocytes with large nuclei and abundant cytoplasm.	Most commonly seen as macrophage-derived in granulomas	
Giant cell	Macrophages with many nuclei as they are formed after ingestion of substance		Seen in foreign body reactions and some granulomatous disease, e.g. ano-genital Crohn's disease
Histiocyte	Macrophages derived from monocytes involved in phagocytosis	Have larger nuclei and more abundant cytoplasm than lymphocytes	
Keratinocyte	Epidermal cell		
Macrophage	A cell derived from the bone marrow that is involved in phagocytosis.		
Plasma cells	The nucleus is eccentric and stippled while the cytoplasm is pale	Common in vestibule as a normal finding	Zoon's vulvitis, syphilis

Special Histological Stains

These stains (see Table 4.3) are sometimes needed to clarify certain structures in the skin and to confirm some types of infection. They can be used to see if there is an increase or decrease in a component of the skin when this is not easily seen on H&E sections.

Table 4.2 Glossary of histopathological terms.

		Clinical appearance	Commonly seen in
Acanthosis	Acanthosis is an increase in the keratinocytes of the spinous layer resulting in a thickening of the epidermis. Histologically there is thickening and fusing of the rete pegs	Seen as thickened plaques	Lichen simplex, psoriasis
Acantholysis	Acantholysis is loss of cohesion among the keratinocytes of the spinous layer with loss of the intercellular bridges	Superficial blisters and erosions	Pemphigus vulgaris, Hailey–Hailey disease, herpes infection
Apoptosis	Necrosis of keratinocytes		Erythema multiforme
Balloon degeneration	Increased intracellular fluid due to injury, which then leads to cell destruction		Herpes infection
Colloid bodies / cytoid bodies	Apoptotic / dyskeratotic cells seen in lower epidermis or superficial dermis		Lichen planus
Dyskeratosis	Cell death with premature and abnormal keratinization of the epithelial cells, below the stratum granulosum; the cells appear small and have an abnormal shape.		Condyloma acuminatum, differentiated VIN and squamous cell carcinoma
Granuloma	A localized aggregation of inflammatory cells often with multinucleated giant cells; they represent a chronic inflammatory response to infectious or noninfectious agents		Crohn's disease, sarcoidosis, mycobacterial infection
Hypergranulosis	Increased number of cells in the stratum granulosum, usually associated with orthokeratosis		Lichen planus, human papilloma virus infections
Hyperkeratosis	Thickening of the stratum corneum, the outer skin layer; the increased keratinocytes may be devoid of their nuclei (orthohyperkeratosis) or retain them (hyperparakeratosis)	Skin thickening, and sometimes looks pale	
Inclusions in cytoplasm	Collection of a substance such a viral protein seen in the cytoplasm		Molluscum contagiosum
Interface dermatitis	Basal layer vacuolation often with apoptotic cells and an inflammatory infiltrate at the dermal-epidermal junction		Lichen planus
Koilocytosis	Superficial cells showing nuclear atypia, surrounded by a large, clear and irregular cytoplasm with clear-cut borders; the nucleus is enlarged (two or three times the size of a normal cell); binucleation is common; koilocytosis is the cytopathic effect of HPV		Pathognomonic for HPV infection
Lichenoid infiltrate	A band-like chronic inflammatory infiltrate of lymphocytes in the papillary dermis, which 'hugs' the basement membrane zone		Characteristic of lichen planus

(Continued)

Table 4.2 (Continued)

		Clinical appearance	Commonly seen in
Orthokeratosis	Hyperkeratosis without parakeratosis; no nucleus is seen in the cells		
Papillomatosis	Increase in size of the dermal papillae, so that there are projections of the epidermis	Undulating epidermal appearance	Condyloma acuminata, acanthosis nigricans
Parakeratosis	Parakeratosis is the incomplete keratinization of the stratum corneum, with the presence of pyknotic nuclei; it is often seen when there is an abnormality in the epidermis and other features are often seen in association such as hyperkeratosis and acanthosis.	Scaling	Psoriasis, eczema
Pigmentary incontinence	Melanin deposition in the dermis commonly seen after inflammation; macrophages may ingest some of the pigment		Postinflammatory hyperpigmentation
Pleomorphism	Pleomorphism is a cell population showing individual morphologic variation, with different size and shape of nuclei; it is seen in association with malignancies		
Pseudoepitheliomatous hyperplasia	Epidermal proliferation that may mimic well differentiated squamous cell carcinoma		Hypertrophic lichen planus, condylomata acuminata, edge of ulcers
Pseudokoilocytosis	Cells mimicking an HPV infection can be seen in different situations (infection, postmenopause, pregnancy); large cells with an increased amount of glycogen may resemble koilocytes		
Spongiosis	Widening of the interspace among keratinocytes due to intercellular oedema without detachment of the cells from each other	Vesicles if severe	Dermatitis
Vacuolar degeneration	Intercellular vacuoles lead to cell damage and death; most commonly occurs at the basal layer		Lichen planus

Immunohistochemical Stains

Immunohistochemical stains (Table 4.4) are most commonly used in diagnosing tumours and to identify certain infective organisms. In the context of vulval disease, they are particularly important in the diagnosis of extra-mammary Paget's disease.

Table 4.3 Special histological stains.

Stain	Cells stained	Uses
Alcian blue	Glycoaminoglycans	Mucin deposition disorders
Congo red	Amyloid	
Giemsa	Nuclei, mast cell granules, Leishmania	Donovan bodies of granuloma inguinale, histoplasma
Gram	Positive and negative bacteria	
Grocott	Fungi	
Iron or Prussian blue	Haemosiderin	
Masson Fontana	Melanin	
Periodic acid-Schiff (PAS)	Glycogen, fungi	Used to identify fungal infection and to highlight the basement membrane
Toluidin blue	Mast cell granules	Mast cell disorders
Thioflavine T	Amyloid	
Van Gieson	Collagen, elastic fibres	Disorders of elastic tissue
Von Kossa	Calcium salts	Calcinosis
Warthin–Starry	Spirochaetes	Syphilis
Ziehl–Neelsen (ZN)	Acid-fast mycobacteria	Tuberculosis

Table 4.4 Immunohistochemical stains.

Stain	Cells stained	Uses
Ki-67	Proliferation marker	
S100	Melanocytes, Langerhans cells, activated macropahges	Melanoma
Melan A	Melanocytes	Melanoma
Smooth muscle actin (SMA)	Smooth muscle cells	
Cytokeratins 7 and 20		Extramammary Paget's disease
GCDFP-15 (gross cystic disease fluid protein-15	Apocrine glands	Extramammary Paget's disease

Other Tests

In situ hybridization is used to identify high- or low-risk human papilloma virus types. Polymerase chain reactions can also be used for viral lesions, atypical mycobacteria and some parasites. They are not used routinely.

Further Reading

Calonje, E., Brenn, T., McKee, P. H. and Lazar, A. (eds) (2011) *McKee's Pathology of the Skin: With Clinical Correlations*, 4th edn. Elsevier, Edinburgh.

Lynch, P. J., Moyal-Barracco, M., Bogliatto, F. *et al.* (2007) 2006 International Society for the Study of vulvovaginal Disease Classification of Vulvar Dermatoses: pathologic subsets and their clinical correlates. *Journal of Reproductive Medicine* **52**, 3–9.

Kurman, R. J., Hedrick Ellenson, L. and Rounett, B. (eds) (2011) *Blaustein's Pathology of the Female Genital Tract*, 6th edn, Springer, New York, NY.

Wilkinson, E. J. (ed.) (1987) *Pathology of Vulva and Vagina*, Livingstone, New York, NY.

5

Investigations in Vulval Disease

As with all disease, the investigation of any vulval problem will depend on the clinical differential diagnosis. The relevant investigations are detailed in subsequent chapters. This chapter discusses the basic investigations that may be needed when diagnosing a patient with vulval disease. Chapter 3 looked at the process of taking a vulval biopsy and histological interpretation.

Before taking any samples it is important to have all the necessary equipment available. Check any special transport requirements or laboratory rules. All samples taken for any investigation must be labelled correctly with the patient's identifying details and the date and time collected.

Investigations for Infection

Bacterial Swabs

Sterile, cotton-tipped swabs (Figure 5.1) are used to collect bacteria. These swabs can be used dry in the vulva and vagina. The tip can be gently rotated in order to obtain the best sample. In the laboratory, the swab is used to transfer the bacteria to an agar plate for culture and identification of the organism and then to establish antibiotic sensitivity where appropriate. Some bacteria need special transport media and conditions to grow and, if a specific infection is suspected, it is best to discuss this with the local laboratory before taking samples, as requirements may vary.

Viral Swabs

Swabs taken for the investigation of viral infection need special transport media. Swabs containing calcium alginate or wood will interfere with the isolation of viruses and are known to be toxic to herpes simplex. The correct swab must therefore be used and these are widely available (Figure 5.2a–c). When taking viral swabs, ideally an intact vesicle should be deroofed aseptically and the blister fluid swabbed, with the swab rotated on the base of the lesion.

Fungal Scrapings

Skin scrapings are used in the diagnosis of superficial fungal infection. A simple scalpel blade or 'banana' scalpel (Figure 5.3) is used to scrape the scaly edge of a suspected fungal infection lightly (Figure 5.4). The scrapings are collected onto dark paper for transport to the laboratory (Figure 5.5).

A Practical Guide to Vulval Disease: Diagnosis and Management, First Edition. Fiona Lewis, Fabrizio Bogliatto and Marc van Beurden.
© 2017 John Wiley & Sons Ltd. Published 2017 by John Wiley & Sons Ltd.

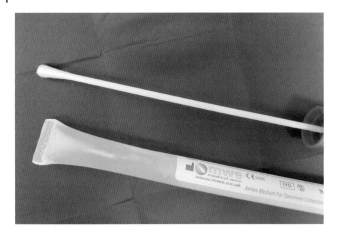

Figure 5.1 Bacterial swab.

(a)   (b)

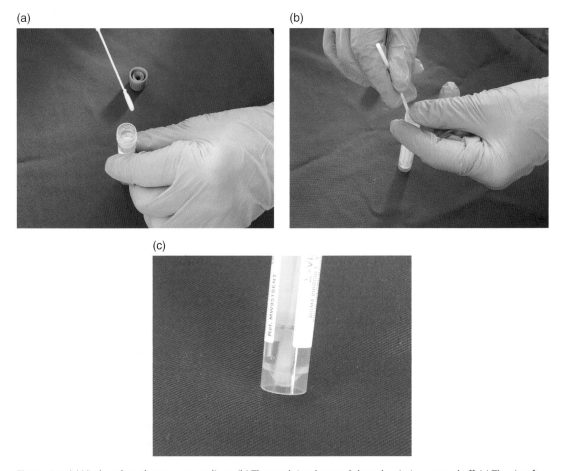

(c)

Figure 5.2 (a) Viral swab and transport medium. (b) The swab is taken and then the tip is snapped off. (c) The tip of the swab is left in the transport medium.

Figure 5.3 'Banana' scalpel used to obtain skin scrapings.

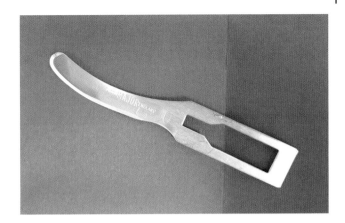

Figure 5.4 The scaly edge of the lesion is gently scraped on to paper.

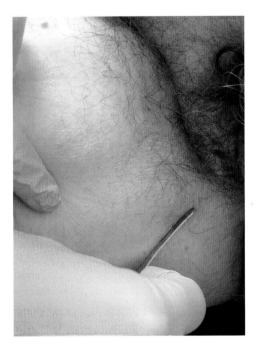

Figure 5.5 Dark paper used to collect skin scrapings.

They can also be collected directly on to a glass slide and covered with one or two drops of 10% potassium hydroxide solution for direct microscopy in the clinic if this is available.

Wood's Light Examination

Wood's light is an ultraviolet light source, which can be very helpful in highlighting certain dermatological disorders. It must be performed in a completely dark room to obtain the best results. Erythrasma fluoresces coral-pink under Wood's light examination. It can also be used to confirm disorders of pigmentation such as vitiligo, where the depigmented areas are more clearly visible.

Serological Tests

Serological tests are useful for some infections and are outlined in subsequent chapters.

Investigations for Allergy

RAST Tests

A RAST (radio allergo-sorbent test) is an *in vitro* test used in the investigation of type 1 allergy. It is safer to use if the patient gives a history of anaphylactic reactions. The current method is the ELISA technique (enzyme linked immunosorbent assay) and it does not use radio labelling as in the original test. This immunoassay measures any interaction between an antigen and the antigen specific antibody. The possible antigens must therefore be considered and appropriate tests requested. No general test will determine the relevant allergen for a patient.

Prick Tests

Skin-prick testing is an *in vivo* method to investigate type 1 allergy. It should be undertaken in specialized allergy clinics where full facilities for resuscitation are available. It detects allergen-specific IgE bound to mast cells. If these are present, this causes degranulation of the mast cells, releasing histamine into the skin, which causes an urticarial weal at the site, which can be measured. Oral antihistamines should be stopped a few days beforehand.

It is generally done on the forearm and a small drop of the allergen is placed on the skin and then a small prick is made at the site through the liquid. A positive control of histamine is used with a negative control of saline. The tests are read after 15–20 minutes and an urticarial weal of 3 mm or more is regarded as positive.

Patch Tests (see Chapter 9)

Patch testing is used in the investigation of type IV allergy. A small quantity of the allergen is placed on Finn chambers (Figure 5.6). Liquid allergens are placed on blotting paper and inserted into the chambers. The strips are then applied to the patient's back and taped in place (Figure 5.7). They are removed at 48 hours and results recorded. They are then reread at 96 hours as some reactions may take longer to develop. An eczematous reaction at the site of application is a positive result (Figure 5.8). A positive result is not always relevant to the clinical problem and can be a reflection of previous exposure to that allergen. Expert interpretation is therefore vital.

Figure 5.6 Allergens at suitable concentration are placed on Finn chambers.

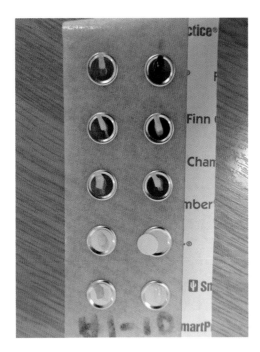

Figure 5.7 Finn chambers taped on back and marked.

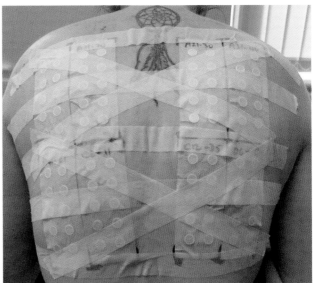

Investigations for Inflammatory Disease

Direct Immunofluorescence

Direct immunofluorescence (DIF) is the gold-standard test in the investigation of immuno-bullous disease. It is sometimes used in connective tissue disorders and vasculitis. It detects auto-antibody/ antigen complexes and uses fluorescent labelled antibodies to bind directly to the target antigen in the skin. There are specific binding patterns in different immuno-bullous disorders (see Chapter 16).

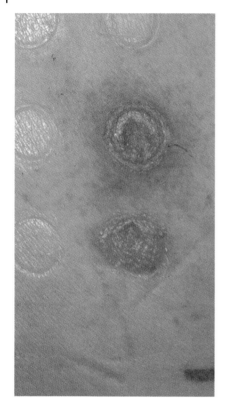

Figure 5.8 Positive patch test reaction – eczematous papule at site of application.

Indirect Immunofluorescence

Indirect immunofluorescence (IIF) has two stages. An unlabelled antibody binds to the target antigen and then a fluorescent second antibody directed against the first antibody is used for detection. It is performed on the patient's serum and can be used to investigate immuno-bullous disease (see Chapter 16).

Imaging Investigations

Imaging is not used widely in the investigation of most vulval disorders but is important in determining the extent and staging of malignant disease. Magnetic-resonance imaging may be helpful in the evaluation of some rare congenital anomalies such as vaginal atresia. It may also be helpful in establishing the extent of hidradenitis suppurativa and Crohn's disease.

Useful Web Sites for Patient Information

British Association for Sexual Health and HIV (BASHH) Sexually Transmitted Infections: UK National Screening and Testing Guidelines: http://www.bashh.org/documents/59/59.pdf (accessed 14 September 2016).

Patient information on patch testing:
http://dermnetnz.org/procedures/patch-tests.html (accessed 14 September 2016);
http://www.bad.org.uk/shared/get-file.ashx?id=113&itemtype=document (accessed 14 September 2016).

Further Reading

Antunes, J., Borrego, L., Romeira, A. and Pinto, P. (2009) Skin prick tests and allergy diagnosis. *Allergologia et Immunopathologia* **37**, 155–164.

Chang, S. D. (2002) Imaging of the vagina and vulva. *Radiologic Clinics of North America* **40**, 637–658.

Fonacier, L. (2015) A practical guide to patch testing. *Journal of Allergy and Clinical Immunology: In Practice* **3**, 669–675.

Odell, I. D. and Cook, D. (2013) Immunofluoresence techniques. *Journal of Investigative Dermatology* **133**, e4.

6

Topical Treatment in Vulval Disease

Introduction

Topical treatment is probably the most important therapeutic intervention in the management of any dermatosis. However, modification to the usual regimens are sometimes required when they are used on the vulval skin. It is important that anyone treating patients with vulval disease is fully aware of how to use these topical treatments appropriately, the potential side effects and how to avoid them. Patient education is vital for the correct use of any topical therapy in order to achieve compliance, obtain the best results and avoid adverse effects. As there is direct contact between the drug and the diseased tissue, the risk of systemic side effects is minimal.

General Principles

A topical treatment (Table 6.1) generally consists of an active ingredient mixed with a carrier or vehicle. This vehicle allows for delivery of the drug into the epithelium and many of the more recently developed treatments contain a vehicle that is tailored to the active drug to achieve maximum efficacy. Therefore, it is important not to modify the specific drug-vehicle system (such as mixing directly with an emollient) as this may significantly alter the delivery and absorption of the active drug. The vehicle must allow maximum stability of the drug and should not have any irritant or allergenic properties. It must also be easy for the patient to apply and must be cosmetically acceptable.

Drugs penetrate the skin barrier depending on their solubility in lipid and water. However, when the epidermal barrier is abnormal in a diseased state, the penetration can increase significantly. There is also increased absorption in flexural sites due to the natural occlusion, which is very important in the treatment of vulval disease. The addition of a chemical such as propylene glycol can greatly increase the penetration as it causes vasoconstriction. This is rarely needed for treatment of the vulva.

Lotions

Lotions are liquid preparations. They include 'shake lotions', where an insoluble compound is suspended in a liquid; for example, calamine lotion. They are easy to apply but are not particularly useful in the treatment of vulval disease.

A Practical Guide to Vulval Disease: Diagnosis and Management, First Edition. Fiona Lewis, Fabrizio Bogliatto and Marc van Beurden.
© 2017 John Wiley & Sons Ltd. Published 2017 by John Wiley & Sons Ltd.

Table 6.1 Classification of topical treatment.

Liquid	Aqueous	Lotions
		Gels
	Alcoholic	Paints
	Emulsions	
Semisolid	With water	Creams
		Emulsions
	Without water	Ointments
	Pastes	

Gels

These are not greasy, are washed off easily and are helpful in hair-bearing areas such as the mons pubis and labia majora.

Ointments

These are by far the preferred formulation for use on the genital skin. They are anhydrous substances and are thicker and greasy for the patient to apply. However, they have an occlusive and therefore protective effect, which is very useful on the vulva where there are several irritant factors that can aggravate the skin.

Creams

These contain both oil and water. Oily cream preparations have a greater moisturizing effect. All creams contain preservatives against bacterial and fungal infection and it is these that often lead to a secondary irritant or allergic contact dermatitis. The differences between gels, ointments and creams is shown in Figure 6.1.

Pastes

Pastes are rarely used for active treatment on the vulva but can be useful when a barrier preparation is required.

Topical Treatments Used for Vulval Disease

- emollients;
- topical steroids;
- antiseptics;
- antibacterials;
- antifungals;
- barriers;
- others.

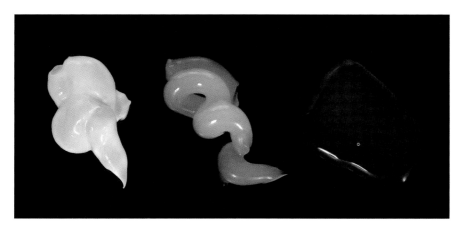

Figure 6.1 Cream, ointment and gel, illustrating differences between the preparations.

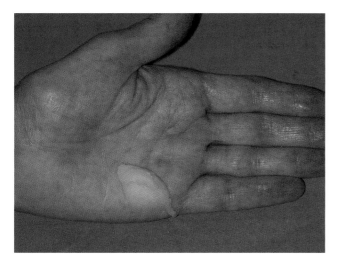

Figure 6.2 Emulsifying ointment used as a soap substitute.

Emollients

Emollients are an important part of the management of any vulval disease. They provide lubrication and moisture when the skin barrier loses its normal structure and function. Patients with vulval symptoms frequently start washing more often in the belief that this will help. The increased use of soap, antiseptics and water can lead to a loss of the natural lipids resulting in a deterioration of the problem. Emollients act to provide moisture and protection at this point.

An effective way to deliver an emollient is to use an ointment such as emulsifying ointment as a soap substitute (Figure 6.2). This can be made into a creamy liquid by rubbing the hands together in warm water. Then this can be used to wash the vulva (Figure 6.3). If patients are also using cream emollients at other times, then the potential for sensitization from excipient ingredients in the preparation should be remembered.

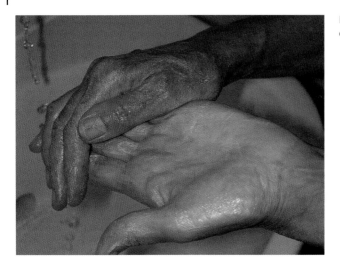

Figure 6.3 In warm water, the emulsifying ointment is made into an emulsion to wash in.

Topical Steroids

Topical steroids have revolutionized the treatment of inflammatory skin disease. However, there has been much publicity about the potential side effects of these treatments and patients are often very worried about using them. The package insert for patients generally states that they should not be used on the genital skin. A thorough explanation of the correct and safe usage of topical steroids should therefore be given to the patient when they are prescribed.

Topical steroids have several different mechanisms of action but it is not known exactly how these take effect. They are anti-inflammatory, vasoconstrictive and immunosuppressive and reduce mitotic activity.

Adverse Effects

The side effects of the excessive use of topical steroids are well known but are uncommon and can be minimized with safe and appropriate use. Once-daily application is now recommended for most cutaneous disease and this is true for vulval disease. There is little to be gained by two- or three-times daily application. Tachyphylaxis is the term used when there is a loss of effect with repeated use of a product. This can be avoided by using reducing regimens of application. In the treatment of lichen sclerosus and lichen planus where an ultrapotent topical steroid is required, it is advised that no more than 30 g should be used in 3 months. Very few patients require this amount. For other diseases, the lowest potency needed for disease control should be used. Once the dermatosis has come under control, it is important that the patient then uses emollients alone and does not keep applying the treatment where there is no disease.

The potential side effects are listed below:

- epidermal thinning;
- hypopigmentation;
- reduced dermal collagen – this presents clinically as striae (Figure 6.4);
- telangiectasiae – these are sometimes seen on the outer labia majora when the steroid is not applied correctly to the inner vulva (Figure 6.5);
- acneiform eruption;
- systemic absorption – this is rare with the small amounts applied to the vulva;
- reactivation of infection.

Figure 6.4 Striae on the thighs after excessive use of a potent topical steroid.

Figure 6.5 Telangiectasia on outer labia majora at incorrect site of application of topical steroids for lichen sclerosus.

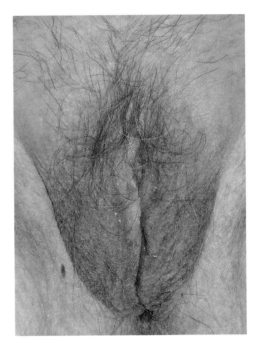

In the treatment of vulval disease, the possibility of reactivating infection with potent steroids is probably the commonest issue encountered in clinical practice. In those with a history of recurrent herpes simplex infection who then require the use of a potent steroid for a dermatosis such as lichen sclerosus, it is worth considering the use of aciclovir prophylactically (200 mg bd) while the topical steroids is required.

If a fungal infection in the inguinal region is not recognized as such, and treated with a topical steroid when mistaken for eczema or psoriasis, the appearances can alter so that the scaly edge is lost. It can resemble a folliculitis and is known as 'tinea incognito' (Figure 6.6).

Topical steroids are graded in potency (see Table 6.2) based on the vasoconstrictor assay, which correlates well with clinical effect. In Europe, a grading system from I (mild) to IV (ultra-potent) is

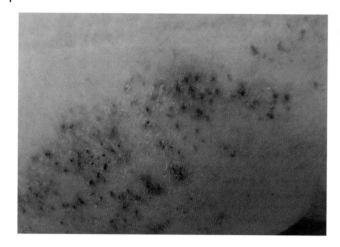

Figure 6.6 Tinea incognito – papules and folliculitic lesions after the application of a topical steroid on a fungal infection.

Table 6.2 Grading of topical steroids (European).

Grade	Potency	Example
I	Mild	Hydrocortisone 1%
II	Moderate	Clobetasone butyrate 0.5% Fluocinolone acetonide
III	Potent	Betamethasone valerate Betamethasone dipropionate Mometasone furoate
IV	Ultra-potent/super-potent	Clobetasol propionate 0.05% Diflucortolone valerate 0.3%

used. In the United States, a seven-point grading system is used, which goes from I (ultra-potent) to VII (mild). Clinicians should be aware of the potency of the treatment prescribed as side effects are generally related to increasing potency.

The steroid molecule is suspended in a vehicle and diffuses into the stratum corneum. The vehicle can alter the potency and ointment preparations can have a greater effect in the genital area as the innate occlusive properties of an ointment increase hydration of the stratum corneum and therefore increase absorption. It has been suggested that a reservoir of steroid exists in the stratum corneum and interaction with other topically applied treatment such as emollients. Preparations that have a higher lipid solubility are generally more potent.

It is often useful to use a combined preparation where the steroid is combined with an antifungal or antibacterial.

For most disease affecting the vulva, an ointment preparation is most useful. However, if there is significant disease in a hair-bearing area, such as the mons pubis, then a gel or liquid formulation may be better. For vaginal inflammatory disease, especially in erosive lichen planus and immuno-bullous disease, the foam containing hydrocortisone acetate used per rectum to treat inflammatory bowel disease is the treatment of choice. It is easy to deliver via an applicator into the vagina and is well tolerated (Figure 6.7).

Figure 6.7 Steroid foam preparation that can be inserted into the vagina to treat inflammatory disease.

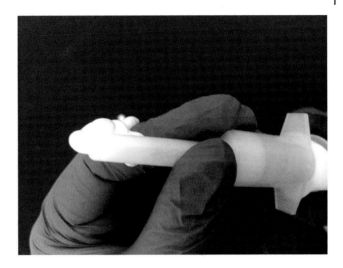

Figure 6.8 Potassium permanganate – dissolve a tablet in warm water to produce a pale purple liquid.

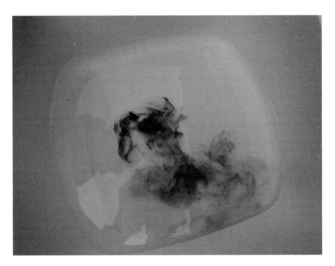

Topical Steroids in Pregnancy

Mild and moderate potency topical steroids are considered safe in pregnancy. There is some evidence of an association of the use of very potent topical steroids with a low birth weight but the quantities used for vulval disease are very small and are not likely to be significant.

Antiseptics

- *Chlorhexidine* is sometimes used in a dilute form as an antiseptic wash in hidradenitis suppurativa but can be irritant.
- *Potassium permanganate.* In an acute, oedematous and weeping dermatitis, potassium permanganate soaks at a 1 in 10 000 dilution can be very helpful. One tablet is dissolved in 3 litres of warm water to produce a pale pink solution (Figure 6.8). Gauze is soaked in this (Figure 6.9) and then applied to the vulva for 10 minutes twice daily. Patients must be warned that this will stain towels and clothing permanently. The skin will stain brown initially but this will resolve as the epidermis renews itself.

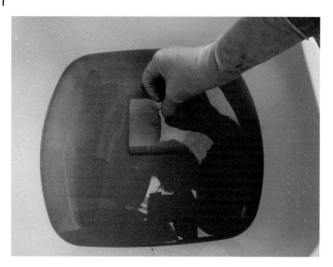

Figure 6.9 Gauze is soaked in the solution and this can be applied to the vulva for 10 minutes.

Antibacterials

If there is significant secondary infection or fissuring then a short course of a topical antibiotic or steroid / antibiotic combination is useful. This should not be prolonged in order to reduce the risk of bacterial resistance.

Topical clindamycin may be used for mild hidradenitis suppurativa and is sometimes used intra-vaginally in desquamative inflammatory vaginitis. Topical neomycin (which is sometimes combined with a topical steroid) is best avoided as it rapidly causes an allergic contact dermatitis.

Antifungals

The imidazole clotrimazole is universally used as first line to treat vulvovaginal candidiasis. It is usually well tolerated but oral treatment is often better if candida coexists with a dermatosis. Other azole preparations are available for use in superficial fungal infections.

Barriers

Barrier preparations contain water-repellent substances such as zinc oxide, silicone or dimethicone (Figure 6.10). They are very useful in protecting the ano-genital skin from the effects of irritants and are generally well tolerated.

Others

Podophyllotoxin
Podophyllotoxin is an antiproliferative drug used in the treatment of warts. It is generally applied twice daily for 3 consecutive days and this three day treatment can be repeated once a week for up to 4 weeks. It is not recommended during pregnancy.

Imiquimod
Imiquimod is an immune response modifier and stimulates the innate immune response via induction of pro-inflammatory cytokines. It has antiviral and antitumour activity and is used to treat

Figure 6.10 Barrier preparation applied to the skin showing the resistance to water.

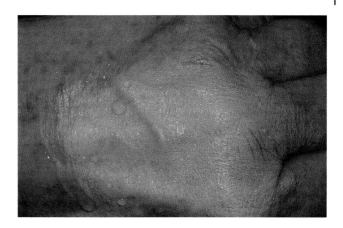

Figure 6.11 Punctate erosions seen with the use of imiquimod.

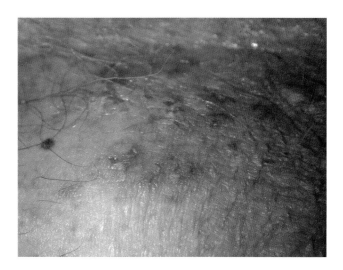

human papilloma virus infection. Unlicensed indications include vulva intraepithelial neoplasia and extramammary Paget's disease (see Chapters 19 and 20).

Erythema and inflammation at the site of application are common. When applied to the vulva, punctate erosions are frequently seen (Figure 6.11). Changes in pigmentation are also common after treatment. Systemic effects including a flu-like illness may occur in about 2% of patients. The frequency of application may need to be reduced to allow patients to continue with treatment. Imiquimod should be used with care in patients with a co-existent dermatosis as this can flare. Rarely, inflammatory disease can be triggered by the use of imiquimod.

Calcineurin Inhibitors

The calcineurin inhibitors, tacrolimus and pimecrolimus are effective anti-inflammatory agents and have been used to reduce the potential side effects of topical steroids in eczema. They have been used in other vulval dermatoses including lichen sclerosus and lichen planus but are tolerated poorly on the vulva with many patients reporting burning on application. There is a risk of reactivating infection, particularly herpes simplex, and concerns regarding the potentiation of malignancy have been raised.

Tar

Coal tar as a weak formulation can be used to treat psoriasis. It has keratolytic and antipruritic properties. The strong tar preparations are too irritant to use on the vulva and must be avoided.

EMLA®

EMLA (eutectic mixture of 2.5% each of Lidocaine and Prilocaine) is a topical local anaesthetic agent sometimes used to reduce the discomfort of injected local anaesthesia for biopsies and surgical procedures on the vulva. It can be irritant and may cause histological changes that can mask the correct diagnosis if the pathologist is unaware of the clinician's practice.

Practice Points

- Patient education in the use of topical steroids is important.
- Once daily application is adequate for most preparations.
- Ensure that you are using the correct potency for the disease.
- Be aware of the potential for a contact dermatitis with any topical preparation.

Further Reading

Chi, C. C., Kirtschig, G., Aberer, W. *et al.* (2011) Evidence-based guideline on topical corticosteroids in pregnancy. *British Journal of Dermatology* **165**, 943–952.

Goldstein, A. T., Thaci, D. and Luger, T. (2009) Calcineurin inhibitors for the treatment of vulvar dermatoses. *European Journal of Obstetrics and Gynecology and Reproductive Biology* **146**, 22–29.

Kai, A. and Lewis, F. M. (2015) The long-term use of an ultra-potent topical steroid for the treatment of lichen sclerosus is safe. *Journal of Obstetrics and Gynaecology* **22**, 1–2.

Lewis, F. M., Agarwal, A., Neill, S. M. *et al.* (2013) The spectrum of histopathological patterns secondary to the topical application of EMLA on vulval epithelium: Clinico-pathological correlation in 3 cases. *Journal of Cutaneous Pathology* **40**, 708–713.

Useful Web Sites for Patient Information

Topical steroids
British Association of Dermatologists:
http://www.bad.org.uk/shared/get-file.ashx?id=183&itemtype=document (accessed 14 September 2016).

Calcineurin inhibitors:
http://www.bad.org.uk/shared/get-file.ashx?id=155&itemtype=document (accessed 14 September 2016).

DermNet:
http://dermnetnz.org/treatments/topical-steroids.html (accessed 14 September 2016).

7

Symptoms in Vulval Disease

A symptom is defined as the subjective evidence of disease or physical disturbance experienced by patients. They then seek medical advice about the cause and its treatment. However, some patients will present without symptoms, but they have become concerned after noticing a change in appearance of the vulva or the presence of a lesion. As outlined in Chapter 2, it is vital to define the reason for presentation and to obtain a clear history of the symptoms and their evolution. Some patients will present with disorders of sexual function, which may, or may not, be associated with a vulval disorder. After assessment to exclude any infection or dermatosis and so forth, the patient will then benefit from referral to an expert in sexual medicine.

Patients who present with a vulval problem generally do so for the following reasons:

- pruritus/itch;
- soreness or discomfort;
- pain;
- dyspareunia;
- discharge;
- change in appearance;
- presence of a lump/lesion.

This chapter will define these symptoms and give the common diseases that give rise to them. Further information can then be found on the specific disorders in subsequent chapters. The lists are not exhaustive as some patients may describe a combination of symptoms and symptoms are subjective. One patient may describe a disease in terms of discomfort and another one could report pain for the same condition. It is helpful when trying to think through a differential diagnosis to group the potential causes into infection (sexually transmitted and nonsexually transmitted), inflammatory, neoplastic and others.

Pruritis (Itch)

Pruritus or itch is one of the most common presenting symptoms in any dermatological condition, but is also frequent in vulval disease. Itch is generally defined as an unpleasant sensation that gives the desire to scratch. Many patients use the term 'irritation' but this is not always synonymous with itch and they may be describing burning, discomfort or pain. It is therefore helpful to ask patients if they want to scratch to bring relief. If they say yes, then the problem is itch. However, if they say no, further exploration of the history is needed to try to define the true symptom.

A Practical Guide to Vulval Disease: Diagnosis and Management, First Edition. Fiona Lewis, Fabrizio Bogliatto and Marc van Beurden.
© 2017 John Wiley & Sons Ltd. Published 2017 by John Wiley & Sons Ltd.

Itch can be exacerbated via central mechanisms or environmental factors. Emotional stress is well known to worsen itch, as will warmth. Patients with vulval disease often report an exacerbation of symptoms in the evening, after a hot bath or in bed. This may be related to increased temperature of the affected area.

The pathophysiology of pruritus is not well understood and no specific skin receptors for itch have been identified. Physical and chemical stimuli can evoke itch and several pharmacological mediators in the skin are likely to be important, such as histamine, prostaglandins and proteases. Scratching can relieve itching for a short time after scratching the skin has stopped, but again the mechanisms are unclear.

Itching may often be replaced with soreness if scratching continues and leads to skin breakdown (excoriation) or fissuring, which is common in vulval disease.

Generalized itching can be related to systemic illness such as renal or hepatic disease or internal malignancy. However, isolated vulval itch is unlikely to be linked to these but may be involved as part of a generalized problem. In this case, the patient should be referred to a dermatologist for appropriate investigation.

Causes of Vulval Pruritis

The term 'pruritus vulvae' is still seen in some older texts but should never be regarded as a diagnosis but as a symptom. The cause of the itching (see Table 7.1) should be established and treated appropriately.

Soreness

Soreness is a very subjective term but is used to describe an area that is sensitive or painful. In the context of vulval disease, this is most often related to those conditions where the epithelium is eroded or broken. The symptoms may be aggravated by micturition or intercourse. Patients may also use the terms 'burning', 'rawness' or 'discomfort'. Causes of vulval soreness are given in Table 7.2.

Table 7.1 Causes of vulval pruritis.

Infection – sexually transmitted	Scabies
	Trichomonas vaginalis
Infection – nonsexually transmitted	Candidiasis
	Tinea cruris
Inflammatory	Eczema
	Psoriasis
	Lichen simplex
	Lichen sclerosus
	Lichen planus – classic and hypertrophic types
Malignancy	Vulval intraepithelial neoplasia
	Extramammary Paget's disease
Others	Urticaria
	Dysaesthetic pruritus – some patients with vulvodynia describe occasional itch but it is never a predominant feature
	Syringomas

Table 7.2 Causes of vulval soreness.

Infection – sexually transmitted	Herpes simplex
Infection – nonsexually transmitted	Candidiasis
Inflammatory	Erosive lichen planus Mucous membrane pemphigoid Pemphigus vulgaris Irritant dermatitis Lichen sclerosus Psoriasis or eczema if fissured Hailey-Hailey disease
Malignancy	Vulval intraepithelial neoplasia Extramammary Paget's disease
Others	Toxic epidermal necrolysis in early stages Stevens–Johnson syndrome Graft versus host disease

Pain

Pain is defined as a highly unpleasant physical sensation caused by illness or injury. It may range from a mild discomfort to severe, where there is a great influence of quality of life and a patient's ability to function normally. Pain is mediated via specific neuronal pathways, which carry the sensations to the brain where they can be modified by many different factors. The quality of pain can be assessed by the SOCRATES or OPQRST-A mnemonics.

SOCRATES (see Chapter 2) is:

S – site (localized, generalized);
O – onset (after vaginal infection, or specific event);
C – character (continuous, intermittent);
R – radiation (back, bladder, rectus);
A – associations;
T – timing;
E – exacerbating and relieving factors;
S – severity.

OPQRST-A is:

O – onset;
P – provoking or palliating factors;
Q – quality;
R – radiation;
S – severity;
T – timing;
A – associated factors.

Causes of vulval pain are listed in Table 7.3.

Table 7.3 Causes of vulval pain.

Infection – sexually transmitted	Herpes simplex infection
Infection – nonsexually transmitted	Herpes zoster infection
Inflammatory	Crohn's disease Hidradenitis suppurativa
Malignancy	SCC Any vulval malignancy may cause pain especially if there is local neural involvement
Neuropathic pain	Vulvodynia – generalized or localized
Others	Lipschutz ulceration Stevens–Johnson syndrome Toxic epidermal necrolysis Postherpetic neuralgia Neuroma

Table 7.4 Causes of dyspareunia.

Infection – sexually transmitted	Herpes simplex infection
Infection – nonsexually transmitted	Candidiasis
Inflammatory	Erosive lichen planus Lichen sclerosus Psoriasis Auto-immune bullous disease Graft versus host disease
Malignancy	Extramammary Paget's disease SCC Any eroded tumour
Neuropathic	Localized provoked vulvodynia
Others	Nympho-hymenal tears Mechanical fissuring

Dyspareunia

The term 'dyspareunia' describes pain with sexual intercourse and may be superficial or deep, with pain felt in the pelvis. In the context of vulval disease, most patients will present with superficial dyspareunia. Women who describe deep dyspareunia must be referred for a full gynaecological assessment. Causes of dyspareunia are given in Table 7.4.

Discharge

It is normal for a woman of reproductive age to have a vaginal discharge, which varies during the menstrual cycle. When oestrogen levels rise before ovulation, the cervical mucus changes from thick to clear and wet, allowing fertilization. However, if the discharge changes or becomes more profuse then further investigation is required to rule out infective or inflammatory causes. Causes of discharge are given in Table 7.5.

Table 7.5 Causes of discharge.

Infection – sexually transmitted	Trichomonas vaginalis Chlamydia Gonorrhoea
Infection – nonsexually transmitted	Bacterial vaginosis Candidiasis
Inflammatory	Erosive lichen planus Pemphigus vulgaris Desquamative inflammatory vaginitis
Malignancy	Vaginal or cervical malignancy
Others	Foreign body Cervical polyps or ectopy Fistulae

Table 7.6 Causes of change in appearance without symptoms.

Infection – sexually transmitted	Syphilis – painless ulcer Warts Molluscum contagiosum
Infection – nonsexually transmitted	Tinea cruris
Inflammatory	Lichen sclerosus (rarely)
Malignancy	Vulval intra-epithelial neoplasia
Normal variants	Vestibular papillae Angiokeratoma
Others	Epidermoid cysts Melanosis Vitiligo Seborrhoeic keratosis Naevi

No Symptoms

There are some patients who, despite a very careful history, do not complain of any symptoms but have noticed a change in the appearance of the vulva. Some causes are given in Table 7.6.

Useful Web Site for Patient Information

International Society for the Study of Vulvovaginal Disease:
http://www.issvd.org/vaginal-discharge/ (accessed 19 September 2016)

8

Signs in Vulval Disease

Clinical signs are the manifestation of disease and are visible findings, such as the presence of a lesion, or are elicited by specific examination, for example touch-provoked tenderness. In some situations, the absence of a normal feature can be very important in reaching a diagnosis; this is particularly important in some of the scarring dermatoses that affect the vulva, such as lichen sclerosus.

It is important to understand the correct terminology in describing lesions (see Table 8.1), as this is helpful in describing cases to colleagues (Table 8.2) and also for documenting change of any disease over time.

Differential Diagnosis Based on Appearance

It is almost impossible to give an exhaustive list of diagnoses purely based on appearance as dermatological disease can vary widely in its presentation. For example, a small epidermoid cyst would be described as a papule but a larger lesion would be a nodule. It will not be until it is excised that it can be established as a cyst as this is not always obvious clinically. Cysts can be felt as firm nodules. A degree of oedema can accompany most inflammatory and infective problems.

The appearance must therefore be examined carefully and a clinical differential diagnosis considered before appropriate investigation leads to a final conclusive diagnosis. Table 8.3 gives a basic list of the common presentations of vulval disorders.

Algorithms

When a patient presents with a vulval ulcer or oedema, there is a wide clinical differential diagnosis. The algorithms in Figure 8.1 can help with investigation and management in these situations.

A Practical Guide to Vulval Disease: Diagnosis and Management, First Edition. Fiona Lewis, Fabrizio Bogliatto and Marc van Beurden.
© 2017 John Wiley & Sons Ltd. Published 2017 by John Wiley & Sons Ltd.

Table 8.1 Terminology of vulval lesions.

Lesion	Description	Clinical example
Macule	Flat area of discoloration <1 cm	Melanosis
Papule	Well circumscribed, raised and palpable lesions <1 cm in size	Molluscum contagiosum
Nodule	Raised, palpable lesion >1 cm	SCC
Plaque	Raised, palpable area	Psoriasis
Vesicle	Raised lesion <5 mm containing fluid	Herpes simplex
Bulla	Raised, fluid containing lesion >5 mm	Bullous pemphigoid,
Pustule	Lesions containing pus which may be infected or sterile	Infected – folliculitis Sterile – pustular psoriasis
Erosion	Superficial loss of epidermis	Erosive lichen planus
Ulcer	Loss of whole epidermis and upper dermis	Crohn's disease
Fissure	Linear split through epidermis and superficial dermis	Vulval psoriasis
Comedone	Plug of keratin stuck in a dilated pilo-sebaceous duct. They may be 'bridged' with an area of epithelium between two lesions	Hidradenitis suppurativa
Telangiectasia	Visible dilatation of small cutaneous bloods vessels; blanch with pressure	
Purpura	Macular lesions containing blood that do not blanch with pressure	
Ecchymosis	Larger extravasation of blood	Lichen sclerosus
Oedema	Diffuse swelling of the tissue	Crohn's disease

Table 8.2 Describing vulval lesions.

Term	Description	Example
Atrophy	Thinning of tissue – may affect the epidermis, dermis or both	Lichen sclerosus
Annular	Ring shaped	Granuloma annulare
Circinate	Circular	Erythema marginatum
Crust	Dried exudate	Impetigo, staphylococcal infection, severe allergic contact dermatitis
Desquamation	Superficial peeling of epidermis	Post-inflammatory change, staphylococcal scalded skin syndrome
Erythema	Red colouration of the skin often with increased warmth, due to increased blood supply to the area	Inflammation, infection
Excoriation	Break in epidermis due to scratching	Eczema, psoriasis, lichen sclerosus
Guttate	Multiple small lesions resembling 'raindrops'	Guttate psoriasis
Induration	Dermal thickening	SCC
Hyperkeratosis	Excess layers of keratin in the epidermis, due to increased proliferation of keratinocytes	Psoriasis

Table 8.2 (Continued)

Term	Description	Example
Lichenification	Thickening of skin usually due to chronic scratching; may be accentuation of the skin markings	Lichen simplex
Reticulate	'Netlike'	Wickham's striae in lichen planus
Scale	Visible flakes of shed epidermal cells	Seborrhoeic eczema, psoriasis
Serpiginous	'Snake like'	Necrolytic migratory erythema
Striae	Linear lesion due to atrophy of the connective tissue	Overuse of topical steroids, Cushing's syndrome
Umbilicated	Small depression in lesion	Molluscum contagiosum
Verrucous	Wart-like	Genital warts, verrucous carcinoma
Weal	Circumscribed area of dermal oedema	Urticaria

Table 8.3 Common presentations of vulval disorders.

Clinical appearance	Examples	
Macule	Malignancy	*In situ* melanoma
	Others	Melanosis Vitiligo Postinflammatory pigmentation Telengiectasia
Papule	Infection	Molluscum contagiosum Warts Scabies
	Inflammatory disease	Classic type lichen planus Early hidradenitis suppuraitva
	Benign lesions	Skin tags Seborrhoeic keratosis Syringomas Pigmented naevi
	Malignancy	Vulval intraepithelial neoplasia Basal cell carcinoma
	Others	Angiokeratomas Fordyce spots
Nodule	Inflammatory	Hidradenitis suppurativa
	Malignancy	SCC Basal cell carcinoma Melanoma
	Others	Epidermoid cyst Hidradenoma papilliferum Bartholin duct abscess/cyst

(*Continued*)

Table 8.3 (Continued)

Clinical appearance	Examples	
Plaque	Inflammatory	Psoriasis Lichen sclerosus Hypertrophic lichen planus Lichen simplex Hailey–Hailey disease
	Malignancy	Vulval intraepithelial neoplasia Extramammary Paget's disease
Vesicle	Infection	Herpes simplex / zoster infection
	Inflammatory	Acute eczema Allergic contact dermatitis
	Other	Lymphangiectasia
Bulla	Infection	Staphylococcal infection Bullous impetigo
	Inflammatory	Bullous pemphigoid Mucous membrane pemphigoid
	Others	Fixed drug eruption Stevens–Johnson syndrome
Pustule	Infection	Candidiasis Folliculitis
	Inflammatory	Pustular psoriasis
Erosion	Infection	Severe candidiasis
	Inflammatory	Erosive lichen planus Pemphigus vulgaris
	Malignancy	Extramammary Paget's disease
ULCER (see Figure 8.1a)	Infection	Syphilis Herpes simplex / zoster infection
	Inflammatory	Aphthous ulcers Lipschutz ulcers (acute genital ulcers) Crohn's disease Behcet's disease
	Malignancy	SCC Basal cell carcinoma Invasive Paget's disease Melanoma
	Others	Drug induced
Fissure	Infection	Candidiasis
	Traumatic	Nympho-hymenal tears (mechanical hymenal fissures) Obstetric trauma Excoriation
	Inflammatory	Psoriasis Eczema Crohn's disease

Table 8.3 (Continued)

Clinical appearance	Examples	
OEDEMA (see Figure 8.1b)	Infection	Candidiasis Cellulitis Filiariasis
	Inflammatory	Crohn's disease Hidradenitis suppurativa Eczema
	Malignancy	Any malignancy, especially if there is lymphatic obstruction
	Others	Urticaria / type I allergy Congenital lymphatic abnormality Venous obstruction Postradiation Cyclist's vulva Pre-eclampsia Ovarian hyperstimulation syndrome

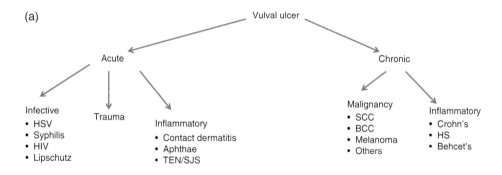

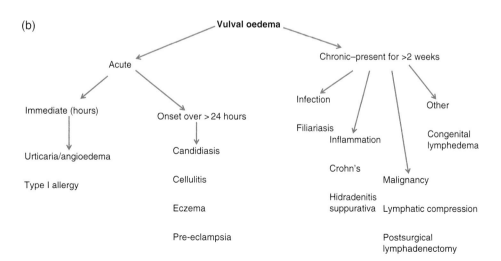

Figure 8.1 (a) Diagnostic algorithm for vulval ulceration. (b) Diagnostic algorithm for vulval oedema.

Further Reading

Bohl, T. J. (2015) Vulvar ulcers and erosions: a clinical approach. *Clinical Obstetrics and Gynecology* **58**, 492–502.

Coutant-Foulc, P., Lewis, F. M., Berville, S. *et al.* (2014) Unilateral vulval swelling in cyclists: a report of eight cases. *Journal of Lower Genital Tract Disease* **18**(4), e84–89.

Lynch, P. J., Moyal-Barracco, M., Scurry, J. and Stockdale, C. (2012) 2011 ISSVD terminology and classification of vulvar dermatological disorders: an approach to clinical diagnosis. *Journal of Lower Genital Tract Disease* **16**, 339–344.

9

Eczema, Allergy and the Vulva

Eczema is a very common inflammatory skin condition with endogenous and exogenous causes. The major symptom is itch. The terms eczema and dermatitis are used interchangeably but 'dermatitis' is often used when the inflammation is caused by the application of an exogenous agent, such as an irritant, or when there are allergic causes.

Eczema does occur on the vulva but there is a tendency to overuse this diagnosis for any itchy, red lesions. It is always important to specify the type of eczema and to differentiate it from psoriasis and candidiasis, which can look similar.

The genital skin is often spared in those with the most common form of eczema, atopic eczema. The three common forms of the disease that occur on the vulva are seborrhoeic eczema, allergic contact dermatitis and irritant dermatitis. These will be considered separately but there are some common principles applicable to all types of vulval eczema.

The pathophysiology is due to a defect in the barrier function of the skin. This leads to the characteristic features of dryness, erythema and inflammation (Figure 9.1).

The histological features of eczema on the vulva are the same as those elsewhere, but may vary depending on whether the condition is acute or chronic. An eczema or dermatitis is characterized by intercellular oedema (spongiosis). In acute cases, accumulation of fluid can lead to the development of small intraepidermal vesicles. Lymphocytic infiltration of the epidermis (exocytosis) is another feature. Secondary infection is common with all forms of eczema and the intense inflammatory reaction seen as a consequence can sometimes cause confusion from the histological point of view. In chronic eczema, the epidermis thickens, with features similar to the hyperplasia seen in psoriasis.

Seborrhoeic Eczema

Incidence

Seborrhoeic eczema is common and the mild form of scaling of the scalp (commonly known as 'dandruff') may affect up to 20% of the population at some point.

Pathophysiology

There is evidence for the role of the yeast organism, *Pityrosporum ovale*, as a pathogenic agent in seborrhoeic eczema. The disease is usually more florid and severe in the immunosuppressed. The histological features can be nonspecific with hyperkeratosis and some neutrophil exocytosis. Yeast organisms are frequently seen on PAS staining.

A Practical Guide to Vulval Disease: Diagnosis and Management, First Edition. Fiona Lewis, Fabrizio Bogliatto and Marc van Beurden.
© 2017 John Wiley & Sons Ltd. Published 2017 by John Wiley & Sons Ltd.

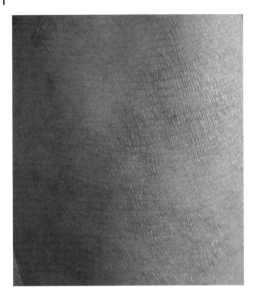

Figure 9.1 Chronic eczema showing inflammation and dryness.

Symptoms

Itching is the most common symptom but soreness and discomfort may occur.

Clinical Features

The signs of seborrhoeic eczema affecting the vulva are often subtle and may just consist of mild erythema on the inner aspects of the labia majora and minora. Superficial scaling may be seen on the rims of the labia majora and keratin debris can build up in the interlabial sulci. It is very important to differentiate this from the 'cheesy' discharge seen in candidiasis. It is important to examine other sites as seborrhoeic eczema rarely occurs only on the vulva. Fine scaling on the scalp and inside the ears will often be found and the axillae and central chest may be involved.

Basic Management

The diagnosis is usually clinical and so a biopsy is rarely needed. An emollient should be used as a soap substitute. A mild topical steroid (grade I/II) can be applied daily for 2 weeks, then reducing in frequency to as required for recurrent symptoms. A combination treatment of a topical steroid and an antibacterial or anticandidal is helpful. Some patients sometimes have recurrent candidiasis, which occurs with eczema and these often need oral anticandidal treatment to allow the inflammatory problem to settle.

General measures, such as cutting the nails, are helpful in all types of eczema. This will at least limit the likelihood of breaking the skin even with significant scratching.

When to Refer

- Doubt about diagnosis or atypical features.
- Failure to respond to treatment.
- Those with coexisting candidiasis.

- The diagnosis is often confirmed by typical findings elsewhere such as scaling of the scalp.
- If severe, think about HIV infection.

Further Reading

Crone, A. M., Stewart, E. J., Wojnarowska, F. and Powell, S. M. (2000) Aetiological factors in vulvar dermatitis. *Journal of the European Academy of Dermatology and Venereology* **149**(3), 181–186.

Useful Web Sites for Patient Information

Dermnetz:
http://www.dermnetnz.org/dermatitis/seborrhoeic-dermatitis.html (accessed 14 September 2016).

British Association of Dermatologists:
http://www.bad.org.uk/shared/get-file.ashx?id=180&itemtype=document (accessed 14 September 2016).

Allergic Contact Eczema / Dermatitis

Introduction

An allergic contact dermatitis can affect the vulva but it is rarely a primary problem and most commonly occurs as a secondary issue when the patient develops a contact sensitivity to a topical treatment or one of its constituents. A helpful clue in the history is that of an acute worsening of symptoms with application of treatment. If the perianal area alone is involved then an allergic contact problem is more likely. Common causes are given in Table 9.1.

Incidence

A high incidence of positive patch tests has been shown in patients who present with vulval pruritus but these may not always be relevant to the problem, and can be a reflection of previous exposure elsewhere. The true incidence is not known.

Table 9.1 Common causes of contact dermatitis on the vulva.

	Example
Topical treatments	Antibiotics, local anaesthetics
Local anaesthetics	Benzocaine
Antibiotics	Neomycin
Preservatives	Parabens, methylisochlorothiazolinone
Fragrances	Propolis
Rubber accelerators	Carba mix
Cosmetics	Nail varnish

Pathophysiology

Allergic contact dermatitis is a type IV delayed allergic response. It occurs after exposure to an allergen and sensitization of the cells of the skin immune system. With repeated exposure, these cells will then elicit an inflammatory response, causing the clinical pattern of an eczema.

Patch Testing (see Chapter 5)

Positive patch tests are often found in patients with vulval symptoms but it is important to investigate the relevance of these to the clinical problem. For example, many patients will have a positive patch-test reaction to nickel but this is usually due to previous exposure and sensitization after ear piercing.

When patch testing in patients with vulval symptoms, it is important to include patch test series other than the basic sets of allergens routinely used, as important allergens relevant to vulval dermatitis may be missed. Preservatives and specific vulval/perianal allergen series should be used and the patient referred to a centre used to dealing with these.

Symptoms

The main symptom is pruritus but in an acute, severe contact dermatitis, pain and difficulty walking and sitting are frequently reported. Symptoms may be intermittent if the allergen is not applied regularly and this may be more difficult to diagnose.

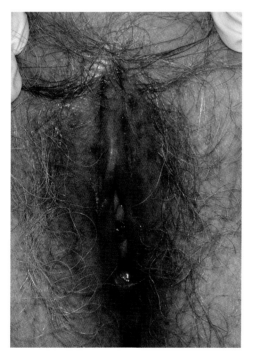

Figure 9.2 Acute allergic contact dermatitis.

Clinical Features

Eczematous areas are seen at the areas of application of the causative agent (Figure 9.2), and may spread to the perianal area and thighs (Figure 9.3). In its acute form, the skin can be severely inflamed and may erode (Figure 9.4), frequently resulting in secondary bacterial infection. Spread to other areas and generalized dermatitis may occur (id reaction).

Basic Management

If the skin is eroded and weeping, the application of gauze soaked in a 1:10 000 dilution of potassium permanganate is helpful to dry out the area (see Chapter 6), allowing the application of a topical steroid. The potassium permanganate is applied to the vulva for 10 minutes twice a day for 48–72 hours. It does not need to be continued for long as it can then cause an irritant problem.

Who to Refer for Patch Testing

Refer if:

- Symptoms worsen or flare with treatment.
- Symptoms spread to other areas, especially thighs or buttocks.

Figure 9.3 Allergic contact dermatitis with extension to perianal area and thighs.

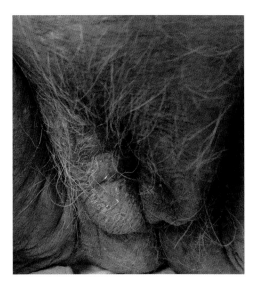

Figure 9.4 Erosions – allergic contact dermatitis to depilatory cream.

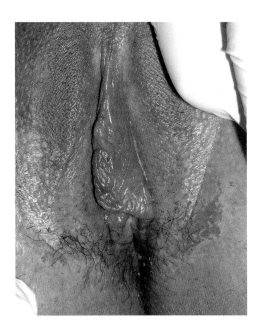

Practice Points

- Think about an additional contact dermatitis if there is a loss of control in any dermatosis.
- A detailed history of all products applied to the skin is needed.

Further Reading

Goldsmith, P. C., Rycroft, R. J., White, I. R. *et al.* (1997) Contact sensitivity in women with anogenital dermatoses. *Contact Dermatitis* **36**, 174–175.

Haverhoek, E., Reid, C., Gordon, L. *et al.* (2008) Prospective study of patch tests in patients with vulval pruritus. *Australasian Journal of Dermatology* **49**, 80–85.

Lewis, F. M., Harrington, C. I. and Gawkrodger, D. J. (1994) Contact sensitivity in pruritus vulvae: a common and manageable problem. *Contact Dermatitis* **31**, 264–265.

Nardelli, A., Degreef, H. and Goossens, A. (2004) Contact allergic reactions of the vulva: a 14-year review. *Dermatitis* **15**, 131–136.

O'Gorman, S. M. and Torgerson, R. R. (2013) Allergic contact dermatitis of the vulva. *Dermatitis* **24**, 64–72.

Useful Web Sites for Patient Information

British Association of Dermatologists:
http://www.bad.org.uk/shared/get-file.ashx?id=113&itemtype=document (accessed 14 September 2016)

International Society for the Study of Vulvovaginal Disease:
http://www.issvd.org/contact-dermatitis-of-the-vulva/-vulva/ (accessed 18 September 2016)

British Contact Dermatitis Society Patient Information on specific allergens:
http://www.cutaneousallergy.org/downloads/ (accessed 18 September 2016)

Irritant Eczema / Dermatitis

Introduction

Whereas an allergic contact dermatitis is specific to the individual who develops a sensitivity to a particular allergen, an irritant dermatitis can occur in anyone who is repeatedly exposed to an irritant substance. Those with a history of atopy are more likely to develop the problem at an earlier stage, and it is more common in those who are overweight. Common causes are given in Table 9.2.

Incidence

Irritant dermatitis is common and is most frequently seen in children presenting with vulval symptoms and also in those elderly women with urinary incontinence.

Table 9.2 Common causes of irritant eczema/dermatitis on the vulva.

	Examples
Topical treatment	Podophyllin
	Imiquimod
	Potassium permanganate
Hygiene products	Sanitary products, panty liners, incontinence pads
	Soaps, detergents
	Wet wipes
	Deodorants
	Lubricants, spermicides

Pathophysiology

The skin in the ano-genital area is prone to irritant problems as it is moist, occluded and the irritant effects of urine and faeces are therefore compounded. An irritant dermatitis occurs when the barrier function of the epidermis is altered.

It is important to ask patients about their own programme of cleaning the area as they will rarely volunteer this information. They will often wash several times a day with products to disguise odour and antiseptics in an attempt to improve their symptoms. Overwashing in this way will undoubtedly make things worse.

Histological Features

The histological features of an irritant dermatitis reveals spongiosis and epidermal cell necrosis. If there is severe disease, full thickness necrosis of the epidermis may be seen. Neutrophilic infiltration of the epidermis may be a feature.

Symptoms

The main symptom is soreness, although some may describe pruritus.

Clinical Features

Diffuse erythema is seen, which affects the outer labia majora, but extends around the perianal area and lower buttocks (Figure 9.5). It is most obvious on the convex areas of skin that have most contact with the irritants and the inner vulva and inguinal folds are relatively spared.

A severe erosive form of irritant dermatitis (Jacquet's erosive dermatitis) was seen in children before the introduction of the modern napkins. This would sometimes develop into a granulomatous lesion called infantile gluteal granuloma and was usually seen on the buttocks. A similar problem is occasionally seen in adults who have urinary incontinence that is not managed well.

Figure 9.5 Irritant dermatitis secondary to urinary incontinence.

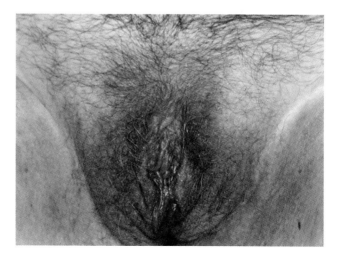

Basic Management

The most important part of management in an irritant dermatitis is to protect the skin. Barrier preparations are therefore vital and need to be applied regularly. These should be continued even after the problem has resolved as once the skin barrier is damaged it has a very low threshold for developing further irritation. An emollient as a soap substitute is useful and, if the problem is severe, a mild topical steroid such as 1% hydrocortisone ointment can help to reduce associated inflammation. If urinary incontinence is contributing to the problem then this needs to be addressed.

When to Refer

- Severe irritant dermatitis.
- Failure to respond to first-line treatment.

Practice Points

- Treat any remediable causes such as urinary incontinence.
- Take a clear history of other products applied to the vulva.
- Advise about barriers.

Further Reading

Bauer, A., Rodiger, C., Greif, C. *et al.* (2005) Vulvar dermatoses-irritant and allergic contact dermatitis of the vulva. *Dermatology* **210**, 143.

Elsner, P., Wilhelm, D. and Maibach, H. I. (1990) Multiple parameter assessment of vulvar irritant contact dermatitis. *Contact Dermatitis* **25**, 20.

Farage, M. and Maibach, H. (2004) The vulvar epithelium differs from the skin: implications for cutaneous testing to address topical vulvar exposures. *Contact Dermatitis* **51**, 201.

Margesson, L. J. (2004) Contact dermatitis of the vulva. *Dermatology and Therapy* **17**(1), 20–27.

Urticaria

Urticaria is a very common problem, and in its idiopathic form, is not considered an allergy. However, an allergic contact urticaria can also exist and so it is discussed here. It manifests as weals or 'hives' on the skin and is due to a release of histamine from mast cells. It generally responds well to antihistamines taken orally. There are various types and the two that can involve the vulva are pressure urticaria and an allergic contact urticaria.

Pressure urticaria is induced with pressure on the skin and can present with acute swelling after intercourse, with or without the use of a condom (therefore excluding a type I allergy, see below) due to pressure on the area. It can be abolished if an antihistamine is taken before intercourse. The patient will often give a history of pressure urticaria at other sites, such as after carrying heavy bags or leaning on an area of skin.

Allergic Contact Urticaria

This is a type I immediate hypersensitivity reaction, with latex and semen allergy being the commonest causes at the vulvovaginal site. It can be complex as occasionally drugs being taken by the male partner or other allergens in the seminal fluid may also cause the symptoms. Semen allergy is rare. The problem is more likely to occur in atopic individuals.

Clinical Features

Immediate swelling of the vulva will occur during or just after intercourse. If it is due to semen allergy, the symptoms will not occur with the use of a condom; conversely, it will not be seen without the use of a condom in latex allergy. The diagnosis can be confirmed by serological testing for latex allergy. It is possible to do intradermal tests on the partner's semen but this is usually carried out in specialized centres.

Management

In pressure urticaria, the use of antihistamines before intercourse can be helpful. A fast-acting antihistamine, such as chlorheniramine, is usually most helpful but the desaturating side effects are sometimes a problem.

In contact urticaria, nonlatex condoms are required if latex is the allergen. If the couple wishes to conceive, then they should be referred to a specialized immunology centre as antigenic treatment of the semen is needed before artificial insemination.

References

Kint, B., Degreef, H. and Dooms-Goossens, A. (1994) Combined allergy to human seminal plasma and latex: case report and review of the literature. *Contact Dermatitis* **30**, 7–11.

Lee-Wong, M., Collins, J. S., Nozad, C. and Resnick, D. J. (2008) Diagnosis and treatment of human seminal plasma hypersensitivity. *Obstetrics and Gynecology* **111**, 538–539.

10

Psoriasis

Introduction

Psoriasis is one of the most common skin diseases and is due to an abnormal proliferation of the epidermis resulting in the characteristic scaly, erythematous plaque. Vulval psoriasis is a common diagnosis in the vulval clinic and studies suggest that psoriasis may account for 5% of those presenting with vulval symptoms. At this site, it is sometimes referred to as flexural, inverse or intertriginous psoriasis.

Incidence

The worldwide prevalence of psoriasis is estimated at 2%. Vulval psoriasis may be found in up to 65% of patients with psoriasis elsewhere but patients are often embarrassed about the disease in the genital area and may not volunteer to describe symptoms at this site unless specifically asked. Vulval psoriasis can occur in isolation, without any obvious disease at other sites.

Pathophysiology

The pathophysiology of genital psoriasis is the same as that elsewhere. There is activation of T lymphocytes leading to an abnormal and accelerated proliferation of keratinocytes. The renewal of the epidermis is reduced from the normal 30 days to about 7 days. The Koebner phenomenon describes the occurrence of skin disease at sites of trauma such as in surgical scars or other areas of injury. Psoriasis is one of the skin diseases that exhibits this frequently and it is postulated that friction, moisture and irritant effects in the flexures may contribute to the development of psoriasis at these sites.

Certain drugs can exacerbate psoriasis and a full drug history is very helpful. Beta blockers, lithium carbonate and chloroquine are known to make psoriasis worse in some patients.

Genetic factors are also involved in the development of psoriasis. Stress and infection are known to be triggers for the onset of disease in predisposed patients.

Histological Features

The classic psoriasiform histology includes regular acanthosis of the epidermis, some spongiosis and elongation of the epidermal ridges and dermal papillae. Intraepidermal neutrophils are seen singly or more typically as small collections. Mitotic activity is marked due to the increased proliferation seen in the condition.

A Practical Guide to Vulval Disease: Diagnosis and Management, First Edition. Fiona Lewis, Fabrizio Bogliatto and Marc van Beurden.
© 2017 John Wiley & Sons Ltd. Published 2017 by John Wiley & Sons Ltd.

Not only are the clinical features of psoriasis lost in flexural disease but the histological pattern is not always characteristic. Spongiosis can be a predominant feature and the histological appearances can be difficult to distinguish from eczema.

Symptoms

The most commonly reported symptom of vulval psoriasis is pruritus. Patients often report that this is worse at night and there may be a premenstrual exacerbation. If the lesions fissure, then soreness, discomfort and minor bleeding may occur. These fissures can be very painful and superficial dyspareunia is common. It can have a significant impact on quality of life and sexual function.

Clinical Features

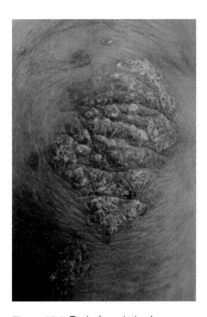

Figure 10.1 Typical psoriatic plaque on elbow showing silver scales.

The classical psoriatic lesion is the scaly erythematous plaque (Figure 10.1). The scaling is silvery in superficial lesions but hyperkeratosis can occur with thickened crusty areas. The classic sites involved are the extensor surfaces (elbows and knees), scalp and ears (Figure 10.2). More widespread involvement affects the trunk and limbs. The face is usually spared. Typical changes occur in the nails with thimble pitting, onycholysis (where the nail plate separates from the nail bed) and hyperkeratosis under the nail plate (Figure 10.3). About 10% of patients will have an associated arthropathy.

Flexural psoriasis may occur in patients with classical psoriasis elsewhere but may also occur as a distinct entity with lesions in the axillae, groins and genital area. At flexural sites, the typical features are often lost due to the moist environment. In patients presenting with vulval lesions it is important to examine other sites as this can often yield useful diagnostic clues.

Vulval psoriasis presents with well defined erythematous plaques, which may become confluent (Figure 10.4). They are usually symmetrical. Scaling is rarely seen but if present will be at the edges of the lesions or on those at the mons pubis (Figure 10.5). Umbilical involvement is sometimes seen with flexural psoriasis (Figure 10.6). The main areas affected are the labia majora and mons pubis (Figure 10.7), but perineal and perianal involvement is common. Extension into the inguinal folds and gluteal cleft is often seen (Figure 10.8) and at these sites, maceration and fissuring is common. (Figure 10.9). This is particularly an issue in those with urinary incontinence. It may occur in obstetrical scars as a Koebner phenomenon.

Some patients have psoriasis and lichen sclerosus together and this can be more challenging to manage and require more regular treatment.

Seborrhoeic eczema and intertrigo can have similar clinical features. Extramammary Paget's disease can often look psoriasiform but is usually asymmetrical and does not respond to topical steroid treatment. Therefore, any disease that does not respond to appropriate treatment should be biopsied.

Figure 10.2 Psoriasis affecting scalp, hairline and ears.

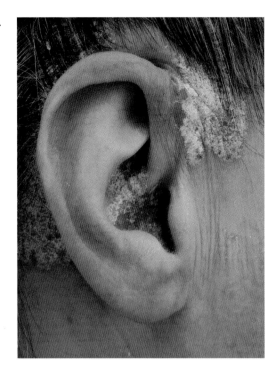

Figure 10.3 Onycholysis and pitting of the nails

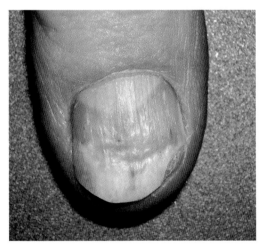

Basic Management

An emollient as a soap substitute, for example, emulsifying ointment, is helpful. If fissuring is a significant problem, a barrier can improve the symptoms associated with micturition. The major treatment for genital psoriasis is a topical steroid and the lesions usually respond to a mild to moderately potent preparation. These can be applied once a day. A reduction in the frequency of application usually gives better results than a sudden cessation of treatment when the problem improves as this often leads to a rebound flare of the disease. Treatment may be needed on an

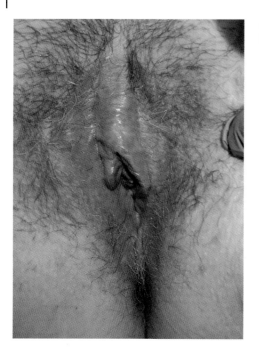

Figure 10.4 Vulval psoriasis – confluent plaques with well defined edge.

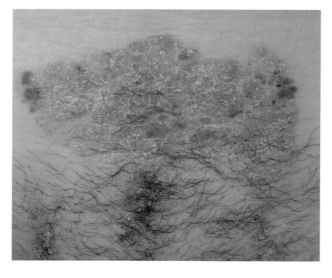

Figure 10.5 Scaling on lesions on mons pubis.

intermittent basis to keep control. Weak coal-tar preparations can be combined with a topical steroid and these are sometimes used in children.

Topical treatments used elsewhere for psoriasis, such as vitamin D analogues and tar preparations, are too irritant to use on the genital skin and should therefore be avoided. Calcitriol or tacalcitol may be tolerated by some patients.

Calcineurin inhibitors (pimecrolimus and tacrolimus) are not licensed for the treatment of psoriasis but can be effective and may be used together with a topical steroid to reduce the amount of steroid required.

Figure 10.6 Umbilical psoriasis.

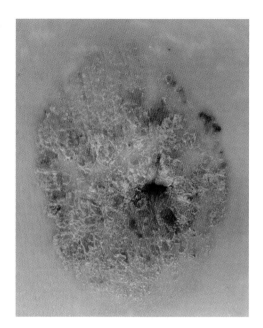

Figure 10.7 Psoriasis with excoriation and scaling.

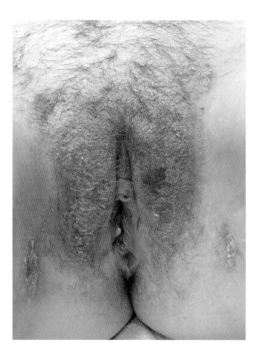

In patients with severe psoriasis, systemic agents such as methotrexate, cyclosporine or an oral retinoid can be considered. Biologic treatments are also used but all of these require specialist dermatological management.

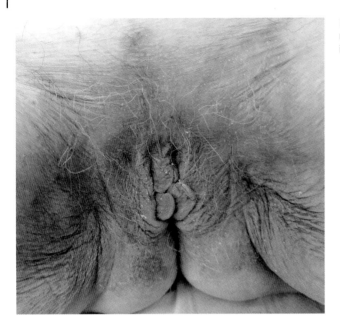

Figure 10.8 Psoriasis affecting the labia majora, mons pubis and extending into inguinal folds.

Figure 10.9 Fissuring in inguinal folds.

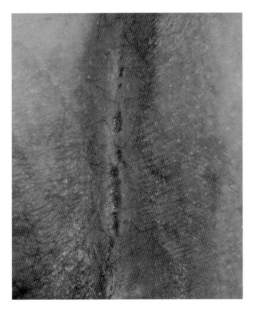

When to Refer

- If the diagnosis is uncertain.
- If there are atypical features.
- If there is a failure to respond to basic management.
- If there is extensive disease, as these patients may require other types of therapy such as systemic or biologic treatment.

Practice Points

- Always biopsy nonresponsive disease.
- Take care with the usual topical treatments used in psoriasis as this needs to be modified in the genital area.
- Intermittent treatment is often required on a long-term basis to keep control.

Further Reading

Kapila, S., Bradford, J. and Fischer, G. (2012) Vulvar psoriasis in adults and children: a clinical audit of 194 cases and review of the literature. *Journal of Lower Genital Tract Disorders* **16**, 108.

Meeuwis, K., de Hullu, J., Massuger, L. *et al.* (2011) Genital psoriasis: A systematic literature review on this hidden skin disease. *Acta Dermato-Venereologica* **91**, 5–11.

Meeuwis, K., van de Kerkhof, P. C., Massuger, L. *et al.* (2012) Patients experience of psoriasis in the genital area. *Dermatology* **224**, 271–276.

Ryan, C., Sadlier, M., De Vol, E. *et al.* (2015) Genital psoriasis is associated with significant impairment in quality of life and sexual functioning. *Journal of the American Academy of Dermatology* **72**, 978–983.

Zamirska, A., Reich, A., Berny-Moreno, J. *et al.* (2008) Vulvar pruritus and burning sensation in women with psoriasis. *Acta Dermato-Venereologica* **88**, 132–135.

Useful Web Sites for Patient Information

The Psoriasis Association:
www.psoriasis-association.org.uk (accessed 14 September 2016)

International Society for the Study of Vulvovaginal Disease:
http://www.issvd.org/vulvar-psoriasis/ (accessed 18 September 2016)

DermNet:
http://www.dermnetnz.org/scaly/genital-psoriasis.html (accessed 14 September 2016)

11

Lichen Simplex

Introduction

Lichen simplex (also sometimes called lichen simplex chronicus) should not be confused with lichen sclerosus or lichen planus. It is a distinct entity that results from chronic scratching and rubbing an area of skin. It is seen at sites that are easily accessible to the patient such as the occipital scalp and lower limb, but the ano-genital skin is frequently affected.

Epidemiology

Vulval lichen simplex mainly occurs in young and middle-aged women. It can start in childhood but is not common in this age group.

Incidence

The incidence of vulval lichen simplex is not known but it is a common condition and accounts for 10–35% of patients seen in vulval clinics. In a series of 183 vulval biopsies of dermatoses, 29% showed changes of lichen simplex.

Pathophysiology

Lichen simplex tends to occur in patients who have a background of eczema or psoriasis, particularly atopic eczema. Rarely, it can occur secondary to fungal infection or other dermatoses and these may not be immediately obvious when the lichenification is severe. In some cases, there is no obvious reason why the pruritus has started. Some authors refer to this group as primary lichen simplex. The role of psychological factors has been postulated and these are important in some patients who may relate the onset of their symptoms to a stressful event.

Histological Features

Lichen simplex is characterized by hyperkeratosis with thickening and elongation of the epidermal ridges. A dermal inflammatory cell infiltrate is usually present and papillary dermal fibrosis is typical.

Symptoms

The symptom is intense itching, which gradually worsens over months and years. Both the vulva and perianal skin can be affected but patients commonly describe vulval pruritus initially, which then spreads to the perianal skin. Premenstrual exacerbation of symptoms is common. As there is no scarring or architectural change in lichen simplex, it rarely causes any difficulties with intercourse.

The itch is intense and patients may wake at night scratching. During the day, the itch may not be so severe but they will often admit to vigorous scratching, which can help their symptoms. Some will scratch until the skin breaks and the sensation of itch is then replaced by discomfort.

Clinical Features

The architecture of the vulva is normal. The major areas affected are the outer labia majora, which become thickened (Figure 11.1). It may also involve the inner aspects of the labia majora (Figure 11.2) and mons pubis. The labia minora are rarely involved but can be thickened if they project outside the labia majora. The vagina is not affected. The skin becomes grossly thickened with a rugose appearance and it is this appearance that is lichenification (Figure 11.3). The skin markings are accentuated and in severe cases, the hair may be reduced because of the trauma of rubbing the skin. It is most commonly bilateral with symmetrical changes but can be unilateral in some cases. In these patients, it will usually affect the side opposite to the dominant hand. Perianal involvement is common (Figure 11.4). Excoriation and superficial ulceration are seen in some cases, especially if the nails are long. Some darkening and pigmentary change are seen in chronic disease.

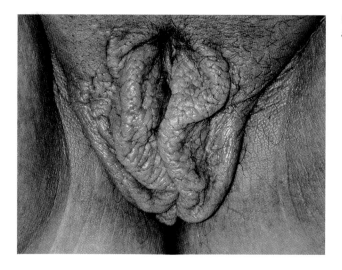

Figure 11.1 Gross thickening of skin on inner and outer surfaces of the labia majora.

Figure 11.2 Lichenification of labia majora and minora.

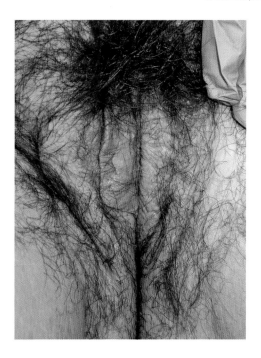

Figure 11.3 Lichenification of labia majora with accentuation of the skin markings and rugose appearance.

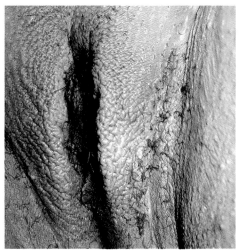

Other sites that are commonly affected with lichen simplex are the lower limbs and back of the neck or scalp. It is important to examine the skin, scalp and nails to look for any signs of psoriasis or eczema elsewhere.

Basic Management

The aim of treatment is to break the itch-scratch-itch cycle and then to deal with any underlying disease. A good explanation of the problem is important. Simply telling the patient not to scratch is unhelpful. Simple measures such as cutting the nails and wearing cotton gloves at night will limit

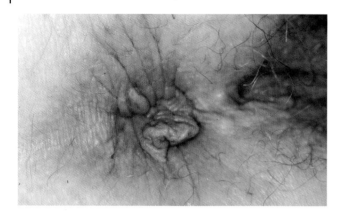

Figure 11.4 Perianal lichen simplex.

the damage from scratching. Any irritants that are being applied to the skin should be stopped. This may require careful enquiry about hygiene habits.

Emollients are useful such as emulsifying ointment, which can be used as a soap substitute. The main treatment is a moderately potent topical steroid preparation applied on a reducing regimen, for example once daily for a month, alternate days for a month and then twice weekly for a third month. The symptoms often respond very quickly but if treatment is stopped abruptly there is usually a rapid return of the pruritus. In most cases, the reducing regimen described above will help. Once the itch-scratch cycle is broken, the problem often resolves. However it is important that the patient knows to apply further topical treatment if there are recurrent symptoms. This can be done on an 'as needed' basis once the problem is under control. In some more challenging cases, topical doxepin 5% cream can be useful. Sedating antihistamines at night such as hydroxyzine 10–25 mg or doxepin 10 mg, may be useful but some may find these cause more prolonged sedation the following day. They should be used with caution in those with cardiac disease. In patients who have persistent lichen simplex it is helpful to check a serum ferritin as iron deficiency anaemia may predispose to pruritus.

In resistant cases, habit-reversal advice and clinical psychological input are often very helpful.

When to Refer

- If there is no response to basic treatment.
- If there is a frequent relapse.
- If there are any atypical features.

Practice Points

- Reduce the treatment slowly to prevent recurrence.
- Review the patient after treatment to ensure no underlying disease.

Further Reading

Ball, S. B. and Wojnarowska, F. (1998) Vulvar dermatoses: lichen sclerosus, lichen planus and vulval dermatitis/lichen simplex chronicus. *Seminars in Cutaneous Medicine and Surgery* **17**, 182–188.

Chan, M. P. and Zimarowski, M. C. (2015) Vulvar dermatoses: a histopathologic review of 183 cases. *Journal of Cutaneous Pathology* **42**, 510–518.

Lynch, P. J. (2004) Lichen simplex chronicus (atopic / neurodermatitis) of the anogenital region. *Dermatology and Therapy* **17**, 8–19.

Useful Web Sites for Patient Information

DermNet:
http://dermnetnz.org/dermatitis/lichen-simplex.html (accessed 14 September 2016)

International Society for the Study of Vulvovaginal Disease:
http://www.issvd.org/genital-itch-in-women/ (accessed 18 September 2016)

12

Lichen Sclerosus

Introduction

Lichen sclerosus (LS) is one of the commonest skin conditions to affect the vulva. It is a chronic inflammatory condition, the cause of which is unknown. It can affect males but is much more common (possibly up to tenfold) in females. Henri Hallopeau described it as a variant of lichen planus in 1889 and, while it is a distinct condition in its classic form, there are sometimes overlap features between the two disorders.

It is important to recognize and treat this condition appropriately as a scarring process can occur leading to an alteration in the normal architecture of the vulva. This, in turn, can cause problems with function, particularly with sexual intercourse and micturition. Once adequate treatment starts and the inflammation is controlled, this process should not progress; hence, it is important to diagnose and treat early.

There is a small but definite risk of malignancy occurring on LS, estimated at about 3–4%. This tends to occur on the hypertrophic or acanthotic types of the disease.

The vulva and perianal area are the most commonly involved and although LS can be found at other cutaneous sites, particularly on the trunk and limbs, this only occurs in about 10% of women with genital disease. Occasionally patients can present with extragenital lesions and it is vital to examine the genitalia as it is extremely rare for the ano-genital skin not be involved in these cases.

Incidence

Lichen sclerosus is estimated to affect 3% of the adult female population and 0.1% of children. However, it is likely to be more common than this as it is often poorly recognized and a proportion of patients are asymptomatic and will therefore not seek medical advice.

The condition has a bimodal peak of incidence. It starts in young girls, usually between 3 and 5 years of age, and then in women after the menopause between 55 and 60. It can start in the reproductive years but this is relatively unusual.

Pathophysiology

The cause of LS remains unknown but several factors have been postulated.

A Practical Guide to Vulval Disease: Diagnosis and Management, First Edition. Fiona Lewis, Fabrizio Bogliatto and Marc van Beurden.
© 2017 John Wiley & Sons Ltd. Published 2017 by John Wiley & Sons Ltd.

Genetic

A positive family history is reported in up to 12% of female patients. There are genetic associations with the DQ7 and DRB1*12 antigens of the HLA system.

Epigenetics

This phenomenon relates to a change in the genome that results in a functional alteration in the expression of a disease. There is no change in DNA sequence. Altered expression of isocitrate dehydrogenase and aberrant global methylation and hydroxymethylation patterns have been shown in vulval LS.

Autoimmunity

IgG autoantibodies targeting extracellular matrix protein 1 have been demonstrated (74% versus 7% controls) and antibodies to the basement membrane zone components BP180 and BP230 are seen in a third of patients.

Hormonal Factors

Reduced dihydrotestosterone is seen in patients with untreated LS and loss of androgen receptors has been demonstrated in genital and extragenital LS. The use of oral contraceptives, especially those with antiandrogen properties, has been shown to be higher in those with LS.

Infection

The role of *Borrelia burgdorferi* has been postulated but there is no consistent evidence that this is significant.

Trauma

Lichen sclerosus exhibits the Koebner phenomenon whereby skin disease occurs at sites of trauma. The extragenital lesions are often seen at sites of friction, for example around the waistline or under breasts or shoulder straps. Lichen sclerosus has also been reported to occur in scars and skin grafts, after sunburn and in radiotherapy fields. It can be seen in episiotomy scars on the perineum.

Role of the Skin Immune System

The inflammatory infiltrate in LS is composed mainly of T cells and there are increased levels of TH1-specific cytokines, all in keeping with an autoimmune phenotype.

Histological Features

The classic histological appearances of LS are a thinned atrophic epidermis and a band of homogenous, hyalinized collagen in the upper dermis overlying a lymphocytic cell infiltrate (Figure 12.1). In early disease, lichenoid changes similar to those seen in LP can occur and may make diagnosis difficult.

It is important to note the thickness of the epidermis as cases where it is thickened and acanthotic may be at greater risk of developing a squamous cell carcinoma and should be followed very carefully.

Figure 12.1 Histology of LS.

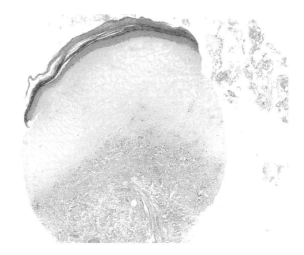

Symptoms

The main symptom is pruritus and most patients describe this as intense, sometimes waking them at night. Minor bleeding may occur secondary to excoriation and fissuring. Some patients may scratch so much that they can induce small areas of ulceration.

If fissuring occurs, discomfort with micturition is a problem. Pain on defaecation and secondary constipation are reported by patients and this is a particular issue in children where constipation can be a predominant and presenting feature.

The introitus can be narrowed due to scarring and this can lead to dyspareunia. If left untreated, scarring can progress, eventually leading to apareunia and problems with the urinary stream which may be diverted and spray on to the thighs.

A small proportion of patients are symptomatic and the disease is discovered as an incidental finding.

Clinical Features

The classic lesion in LS is a white plaque, which can be atrophic (Figure 12.2) or sclerotic (Figure 12.3). At extragenital sites, follicular delling is a feature and if the areas are atrophic, the surface of the skin is said to look like wrinkled cigarette paper. Ecchymosis or purpura is a pathognomonic feature and can be seen at genital and extragenital sites (Figure 12.4).

On the vulva, early lesions are seen as white papules. These are usually symmetrical but then coalesce to form white plaques (Figure 12.5). These are most commonly found on the inner aspects of the labia majora, labia minora, perineum and clitoral hood. Perianal lesions are seen in about 30% of women (Figure 12.6) and when present give rise to a 'figure-of-eight' appearance. Localized disease may occur and the clitoral hood is a very common site for this.

Ecchymosis is a common feature and in some patients may be widespread on the vulva (Figure 12.7). The appearance of these lesions may be distressing to patients but is not concerning and usually responds well to treatment. Excoriation and superficial ulceration may be seen, which is attributable to scratching. In children, bullous lesions may occur, but these are rare in adults. In some patients

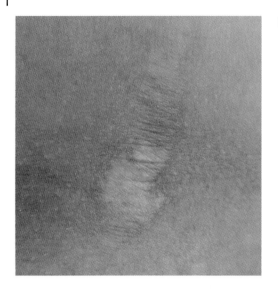

Figure 12.2 Atrophic extragenital LS.

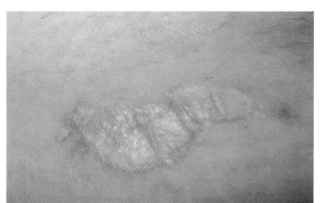

Figure 12.3 Sclerotic extragenital LS.

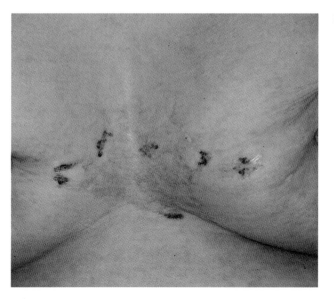

Figure 12.4 Ecchymosis in extragenital LS.

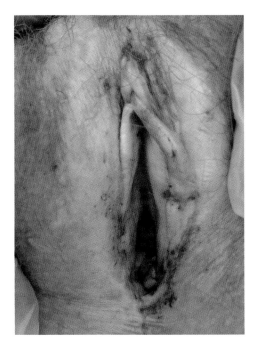

Figure 12.5 Symmetrical white plaques on labia majora.

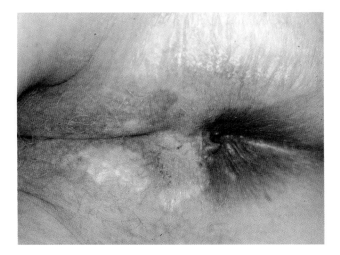

Figure 12.6 Perianal LS.

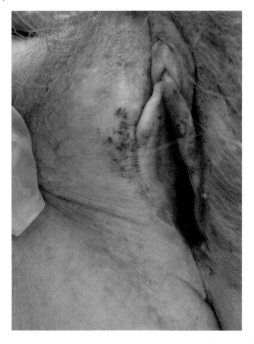

Figure 12.7 Ecchymosis (purpura) can be widespread in some patients.

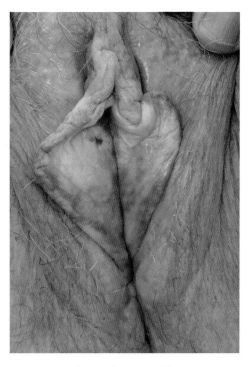

Figure 12.8 Sclerotic plaques on labia minora.

the areas are very sclerotic and oedematous (Figure 12.8). Postinflammatory hyperpigmentation is common and can be marked (Figures 12.9 and 12.10). These features are the same in prepubertal disease (Figure 12.11).

As the disease progresses, the normal anatomical features of the vulva are changed. The labia minora may be partially or completely resorbed and then fuse anteriorly and/or posteriorly (Figure 12.12). The clitoral hood becomes tethered down so that it is not freely retracted. Eventually this can seal over with burial of the clitoris (Figure 12.13). A clitoral pseudocyst can sometimes develop in this situation.

Lichen sclerosus does not affect the vagina except in the rare circumstance where a prolapse of the vagina mucosa occurs. If this then becomes keratinized, LS can occur on this mucosa (Figure 12.14).

Some patients develop thickened lesions on the vulva. They may become hyperkeratotic and are often more resistant to treatment (Figure 12.15)

The main differential diagnosis in LS is that of lichen planus but lichen simplex, psoriasis and vulval intraepithelial neoplasia can also sometimes have similar features. In children, where bullous lesions

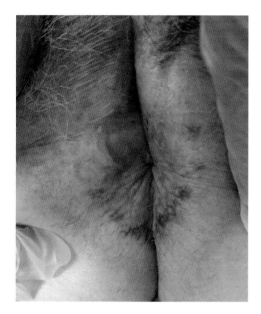

Figure 12.9 Postinflammatory hyperpigmentation in LS.

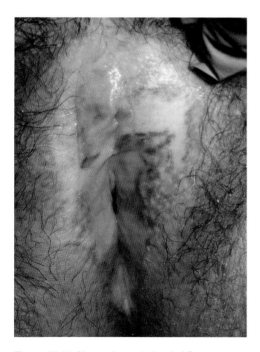

Figure 12.10 Hyperpigmentation in LS.

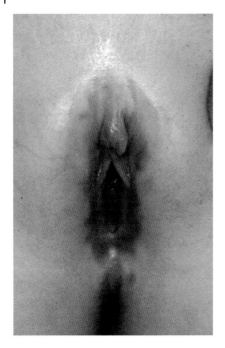

Figure 12.11 Pre-pubertal LS.

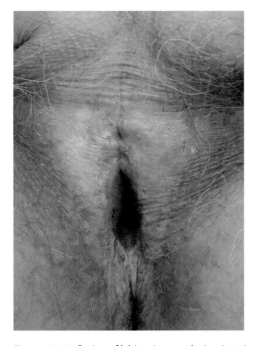

Figure 12.12 Fusion of labia minora reducing introitus.

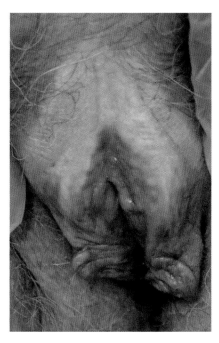

Figure 12.13 Sealing clitoral hood and burial of clitoris.

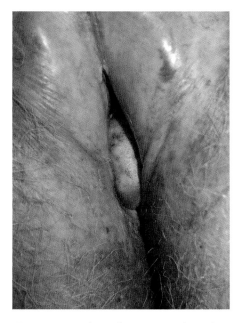

Figure 12.14 Lichen sclerosus on prolapsed vaginal mucosa.

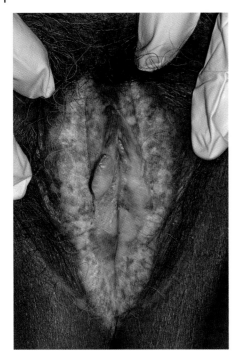

Figure 12.15 Acanthotic disease.

can occur, the rare chronic bullous dermatosis of childhood should be considered as a differential diagnosis. A biopsy should always be taken if there is clinical doubt about the diagnosis or there are atypical features.

Associated Disease

There is a definite association with autoimmune disorders in about 30% of patients with LS and there may also be a positive family history of autoimmunity. The most frequent autoimmune disease seen in these patients is thyroid disease, usually hypothyroidism. Vitiligo, alopecia areata, pernicious anaemia, primary biliary cirrhosis and others are also reported.

Some patients have anogenital psoriasis and LS (Figure 12.16). This combination is sometimes more difficult to control.

Risk of Malignancy

The risk of developing a squamous cell carcinoma on a background of lichen sclerosus is about 4%. (Figure 12.17). However, in well controlled disease, this risk appears to be much less but there is no current evidence to suggest that it is abolished by treatment. Any patient with a significant change in symptoms, or with the development of a nonhealing ulcer or nodule, should be reviewed urgently.

Figure 12.16 Lichen sclerosus and psoriasis can coexist.

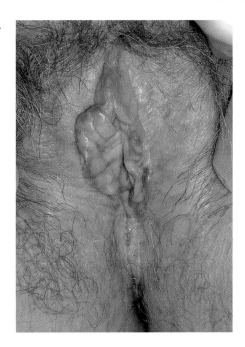

Figure 12.17 Squamous cell carcinoma developing on LS.

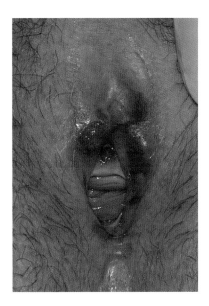

Differentiated vulval intraepithelial neoplasia (dVIN) is often seen at the edge of a squamous cell carcinoma (see Chapter 19). In patients with unstable disease with a poor response to topical steroids applied correctly, there should be a low threshold to biopsy any superficially ulcerated or excoriated lesions. The pathologist must be made aware of the suspicion of dVIN as the histological features are subtle. If it is seen on biopsies, these areas should be excised, and the patient carefully monitored.

Basic Management

The aims of treatment are to control symptoms and to preserve function. The pallor of LS will often remain even in well controlled and quiescent disease. As a general measure, an emollient used as a soap substitute is helpful.

The first-line management for LS, in adults and children, is an ultrapotent topical steroid. Clobetasol propionate 0.05% is most frequently prescribed and the ointment preparation is generally well tolerated. A 3-month course of treatment on a reducing regimen – once a day for one month, alternate days for the second month and then twice weekly for the third month – is recommended. After this it can be used once a day as needed. Mometasone furoate, betamethasone dipropionate and fluandrolone are alternatives as some patients rarely become sensitized to the steroid or one of its component ingredients.

Calcineurin inhibitors (pimecrolimus and tacrolimus) have been reported to be helpful but should not be used first line and there are concerns about the reactivation of infection and the development of malignancy with their use. The efficacy of a potent topical steroid has been shown to be superior to tacrolimus and pimecrolimus.

In general patients can use treatment as required to control symptoms but, for those with more active disease, continued treatment once or twice weekly can be useful to maintain good control.

There is no role of the use of topical testosterone in the management of LS. Surgery should only be considered in two situations. Firstly, if there is any evidence of differentiated vulval intraepithelial neoplasia or squamous cell carcinoma this must be excised. Secondly, if there is severe scarring with functional sequelae, this may need division of adhesions to allow normal micturition and to improve sexual function.

Other treatments that have been used include phototherapy, retinoids and photodynamic therapy but these are rarely necessary if topical steroids are used correctly and should only be undertaken under specialist supervision.

Follow Up

Patients should be followed up to ensure their disease is well controlled. For those with uncomplicated disease that responds well to treatment, they can be discharged from the clinic with good patient information and advice about treatment and signs to look for. For patients who require regular treatment, or who have hyperkeratotic disease, continued monitoring is needed. Any patient with a history of vulval intraepithelial neoplasia or squamous cell carcinoma and LS should be kept under specialist review.

When to Refer

- If the diagnosis is uncertain.
- If there is failure to respond to first-line treatment.
- If there are atypical features.
- Any patient with a history of differentiated vulval intraepithelial neoplasia or squamous cell carcinoma should be under the care of a specialist clinic.

Practice Points

- Always biopsy atypical disease or where is lack of response to treatment
- Ensure that patients who do not respond to first-line treatment are compliant with the treatment and are using it correctly. It is also important to exclude a secondary problem such as a superadded infection like candidiasis or an allergic contact dermatitis response to treatment but this is rare. A clue is that the problem becomes worse after application and there may be an eczematous rash extending on to the thighs.
- Think about vulval pain in those with well controlled disease but who complain of pain. In this situation, increasing the potency of the topical steroid or changing to another will not help and they need to be treated for vulvodynia.
- Patients with hyperkeratotic or acanthotic disease should be monitored carefully.

Further Reading

Chi, C. C., Kitschig, G., Baldo, M. *et al.* (2011) Topical interventions of genital lichen sclerosus (Review). *Cochrane Database of Systematic Reviews* **7**(12) (Art. No.: CD008240).

Fistarol, S. K. and Itin, P. H. (2013) Diagnosis and treatment of lichen sclerosus. An update. *American Journal of Clinical Dermatology* **14**, 27–47.

Lewis, F. M. (2014) Lichen sclerosus, in *The Treatment of Skin Disease*, 4th edn (ed. M. G. Lebwohl). Elsevier, Philadelphia, PA, pp. 399–401.

Neill, S. M., Lewis, F. M., Tatnall, F. M. and Cox, N. H. (2010) British Association of Dermatologists' guidelines for the management of lichen sclerosus 2010. *British Journal of Dermatology* **163**, 672–682.

Useful Web Sites for Patient Information

Association for Lichen Sclerosus and Vulval Health:
www.lichensclerosus.org (accessed 14 September 2016).

BASHH guidelines on vulval conditions:
http://www.bashh.org/documents/2014_vulval_guidelines%20Final.pdf (accessed 14 September 2016)

British Association of Dermatologists patient information:
http://www.bad.org.uk/shared/get-file.ashx?id=291&itemtype=document (accessed 14 September 2016)

DermNet:
http://dermnetnz.org/immune/lichen-sclerosus.html (accessed 14 September 2016)

International Society for Study of Vulvovaginal Disease:
http://www.issvd.org/vulvar-lichen-sclerosus/ (accessed 18 September 2016)
http://www.issvd.org/vulvar-lichen-sclerosus-in-children/ (accessed 18 September 2016)

13

Lichen Planus

Introduction

Lichen planus (LP) is another dermatosis that specifically affects the vulva but, unlike lichen sclerosus, it can affect many other cutaneous and mucosal sites and has a wide variety of clinical types and presentations.

Epidemiology

Lichen planus is slightly more common in females (approximately 55% of cases) than males and most commonly starts in the 40s and 50s. Vulval LP is rare in children.

Incidence

The incidence of vulval LP is unknown. In one series of 3350 women seen in a vulval clinic, 3.7% had LP on histology and the erosive type of LP was seen in 17.6% of these. Most patients who are diagnosed with cutaneous LP will be asked about, and examined for, oral disease but this is often not the case for genital lesions. Over half of women who present with cutaneous LP have vulval involvement with the disease but may be asymptomatic and so, if not specifically examined, this group may be missed.

Pathophysiology

It is likely that LP is a T-lymphocyte-mediated inflammatory disorder but specific antigens have not been identified. On the oral mucosa, lichenoid reactions are seen adjacent to metal amalgam fillings, which resolve if the filling is removed, suggesting an antigen-antibody interaction. The lichenoid form of graft versus host disease has features that are indistinguishable from those of LP on the mucosa. A link between LP and hepatitis C infection has been demonstrated in some populations in southern Europe but not in others and there is no link in northern Europe.

An association with other autoimmune diseases such as thyroid disease, pernicious anaemia, vitiligo and alopecia areata can be seen in patients with LP. A genetic link has been demonstrated with the vulvo-vaginal-gingival subtype of erosive LP.

A Practical Guide to Vulval Disease: Diagnosis and Management, First Edition. Fiona Lewis, Fabrizio Bogliatto and Marc van Beurden.

Histological Features

The typical features of LP are a thickened epidermis with a prominent granular cell layer and irregular 'saw-tooth' acanthosis. Under the basal layer, a dense dermal inflammatory infiltrate consisting mainly of T lymphocytes occurs in a bandlike pattern (Figure 13.1). Basal cell liquefactive degeneration with the formation of colloid bodies (apoptotic basal cells) is typical. Pigmentary incontinence is common. Some atypia can occur in the basal layer as the cells regenerate and it is important not to mistake this for intraepithelial neoplasia.

These classical features are most likely to be evident in classic and hypertrophic LP. The appearances may be altered on mucosal surfaces and this is a particular issue with erosive LP where the epidermis is lost and the pathologist may report a nonspecific inflammation related to the dense inflammatory cell infiltrate. The best area to take the biopsy if erosive LP is suspected is across the edge of an erosion. Plasma cells may be frequent in genital, LP especially if the biopsy is taken from the vestibule.

Clinical Features of Lichen Planus

The classic lesions of LP are violaceous papules with a white network on the surface, known as Wickham's striae (Figure 13.2). The cutaneous lesions are typically found on the flexor aspects of the wrists, lower limbs and trunk. Flexural lesions affecting the axillae, inframammary areas and inguinal folds can occur with or without lesions elsewhere. The lesions can be very itchy and typically leave significant postinflammatory hyperpigmentation as they resolve, especially in the flexures (Figure 13.3).

Scarring alopecia may be patchy, generalized or in a specific frontal pattern known as frontal fibrosing alopecia or Kossard's disease. A destructive nail dystrophy is seen in some patients.

Oral lesions are frequently picked up at routine dental examinations as they may be asymptomatic and the only manifestation of the disease. Reticulate lesions affect the buccal mucosal surface, gingival margins (Figure 13.4) and tongue.

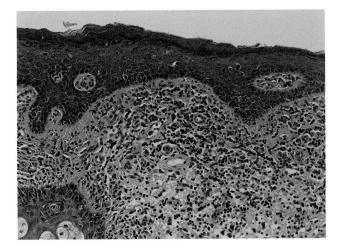

Figure 13.1 Typical histological features of LP.

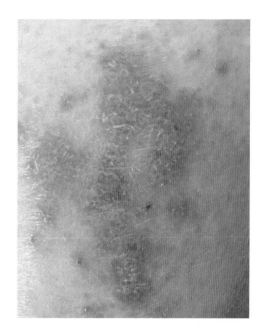

Figure 13.2 Plaque of lichen planus with Wickham's striae on the surface.

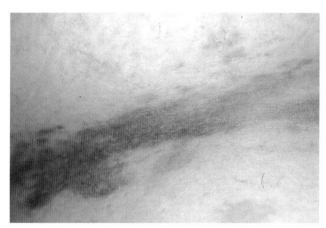

Figure 13.3 Postinflammatory hyperpigmentation in inguinal fold.

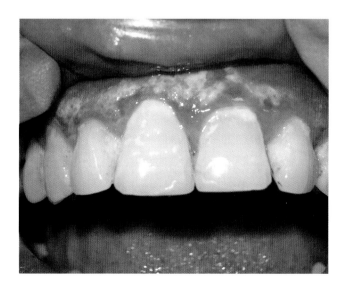

Figure 13.4 Lichen planus affecting gingival margins.

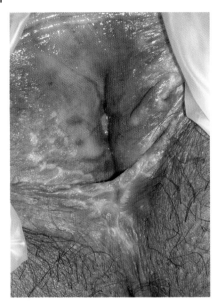

Figure 13.5 Classic type of vulval LP with Wickham's striae.

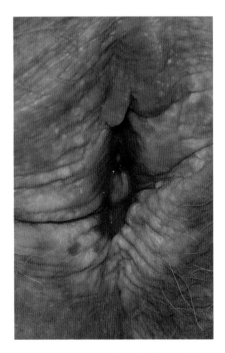

Figure 13.6 Hypertrophic LP affecting labia majora.

Vulval Lichen Planus

There are three forms of LP that affect the vulva – classic, hypertrophic and erosive.

Classic LP

This type may be seen with cutaneous LP but can occur in isolation. It is often pruritic. Papules and Wickham's striae are seen in the interlabial sulci, labia majora, labia minora (Figure 13.5) and over the clitoral hood. There is rarely any architectural change and it can resolve spontaneously.

Hypertrophic LP

Hypertrophic LP is the least common form seen but is important as it has the greatest risk of malignant change. It is symptomatic with severe pruritus being the major problem. It mainly affects the labia majora (Figure 13.6), perineal and perianal areas. The plaques can thicken and may sometimes mimic a tumour.

Erosive LP

Erosive LP is the commonest form to affect the vulva and is important to manage appropriately as the scarring that can result from late diagnosis and inadequate treatment can be extensive, with a significant impact on sexual function and quality of life. Early treatment and careful follow up can prevent this.

The lesions are sore, with pain on sexual intercourse being a frequent presenting symptom. The erosions usually start at the fourchette, extending into the vestibule and the inner aspects of the labia minora (Figure 13.7). The edge of the erosions has a scalloped and lacy appearance. Other sites that can be affected by erosive LP are given in Table 13.1.

Scarring is common with loss of the labia minora, then anterior and posterior fusion leading to a narrowing of the introitus. The clitoris is sealed under the fused clitoral hood (Figure 13.8).

A subtype of erosive LP is the vulvo-vaginal-gingival syndrome (VVG). Vaginal lesions are erosive and friable and can present with a bloodstained discharge. Any patient with vulval LP must be examined for vaginal disease as these patients develop vaginal synechiae and stenosis easily.

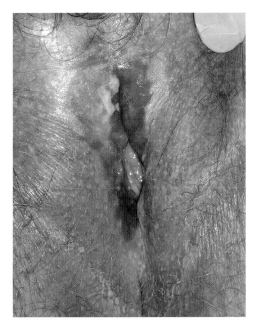

Figure 13.7 Erosive LP.

Table 13.1 Other sites that can be affected by erosive LP.

	Symptoms	Signs
Perianal skin	Pain on defaecation, occasional itching	Erosions, erythema that may extend into anal canal
Urethra	Difficulty starting the stream, frequent urinary tract infections	Erythema and erosions around urethral meatus
Lacrimal duct	Excessive watering of the eyes	White scarring around lacrimal duct (Figure 13.9)
External auditory meatus	Hearing loss	Inflammation seen on otoscopy
Oesophagus	Dysphagia, feeling of food 'sticking' .	Friable erosions visible on endoscopy. Increased risk of oesophageal malignancy

Risk of Malignancy

Squamous cell carcinoma can occur on vulval LP (Figure 13.10) and the hypertrophic type is probably most at risk of this. The risk is not well quantified but is probably about 3–4%, similar to that of lichen sclerosus.

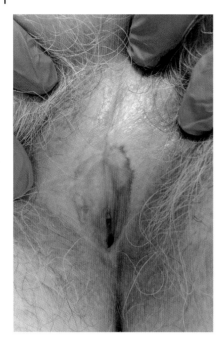

Figure 13.8 Scarring in erosive LP.

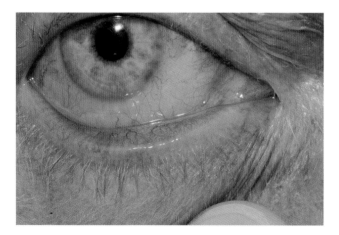

Figure 13.9 Scarring around lacrimal duct in lichen planus.

Basic Management

The aims of treatment in LP are to improve symptoms and prevent scarring and therefore maintain function. Vestibular erythema may remain even when the erosions have healed. Patients with erosive LP should be managed in a specialized vulval clinic where there is multidisciplinary engagement with other specialists (e.g. gastroenterologists, ENT surgeons, ophthalmologists, urologists) who are familiar with treating the disease at other sites.

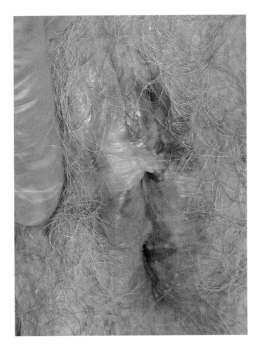

Figure 13.10 Squamous cell carcinoma in LP – eroded tumour left labium majus.

The first-line management of all types of LP is an ultrapotent topical steroid. A three-month course of clobetasol propionate 0.05% ointment may be all that is required for the classic type of the disease. Patients with the erosive and hypertrophic types are very likely to require ongoing treatment for good disease control. It is important to educate the patient about the correct and safe use of topical treatments at the site.

The calcineurin inhibitors tacrolimus and pimecrolimus have been shown to be helpful in vulval LP but the effects are often temporary. Their use is also limited by poor tolerability as they sting on application. There are also some concerns about a possible increased risk of malignancy and reactivation of infection.

Treatment of vaginal LP is important and one of the easiest ways to deliver a topical steroid into the vagina is with the hydrocortisone acetate foam used to treat inflammatory bowel disease (see Chapter 6). One applicator of foam is inserted into the vagina at night for 2 weeks and then the frequency is reduced to once or twice weekly with regular follow up to assess response. If synechiae and stenosis has developed, then this will require surgery. This needs to be done by someone experienced in the procedure and postoperative care is vital as restenosis will occur quickly if topical steroids are not used within 24-48 hours of surgery to treat the inflammatory disease.

When to Refer

- Patients with erosive LP or VVG syndrome.
- Other types where there is a failure to respond to first-line management.
- Vaginal involvement or severe vulval scarring.
- Any patient where a squamous cell carcinoma is suspected.

Practice Points

- Examine for vaginal disease.
- Check other potential sites of involvement.

Further Reading

Lewis, F. M. and Bogliatto, F. (2013) Erosive vulval lichen planus – a diagnosis not to be missed: a clinical review. *European Journal of Obstetrics and Gynecology and Reproductive Biology* **171**, 214–219.

Pelisse, M., Leibowitch, M., Sedel, D. and Hewitt, J. (1982) Un nouveau syndrome vulvo-vagino-gingival. Lichen plan erosive plurimuqueux. *Annales de dermatologie et de vénéréologie* **109**, 797–798.

Useful Web Sites for Patient Information

DermNet:
http://www.dermnetnz.org/site-age-specific/erosive-lichen-planus.html (accessed 14 September 2016)

International Society for the Study of Vulvovaginal Disease:
http://www.issvd.org/vulvar-lichen-planus/ (accessed 18 September 2016)

UK Lichen Planus Support Group:
www.uklp.org.uk/ (accessed 14 September 2016)

14

Hidradenitis Suppurativa and Crohn's Disease

Hidradenitis Suppurativa

Introduction

Hidradenitis suppurativa (HS) is a chronic inflammatory disease mainly occurring in areas where apocrine glands are commonly situated – the axillae, inguinal folds, perineum, genitalia and breasts. It is characterized by recurrent inflammatory nodules, abscesses and sinus formation with scarring. In some patients the clinical features may overlap with those of Crohn's disease and painful axillary lesions are reported in 17% of those with Crohn's disease.

Epidemiology

Hidradenitis suppurativa is more common in women and usually starts after puberty. The disease may be most active among individuals in their 30s and 40s. Genital and inguinal lesions are more common in females. Risk factors include smoking and obesity.

Incidence

The global prevalence is 1% but the point prevalence can be up to 4% in young females. An autosomal dominant mode of inheritance has been identified and many patients will give a positive family history of HS, acne or pilonidal sinuses.

Pathophysiology

The exact pathogenesis is not clear but the evidence points to follicular inflammation, which then progresses to scarring and sinus tract formation. The main pathology is inflammation but infection is very common as a secondary problem.

Histological Features

The diagnosis is usually made on the classic clinical features. Histological examination shows sinus tracts lined with granulation tissue and squamous epithelium and surrounded by fibrosis. Abscess formation and suppuration are common and this suppuration can extend deep into the connective tissue with an associated marked inflammatory infiltrate.

Symptoms

Pain is usually the most reported symptom. When the lesions discharge, this can be malodorous and offensive. In females, there is often a premenstrual flare of symptoms. Hidradenitis suppurativa has a significant negative effect on quality of life and is reported to have more of an impact than severe psoriasis and eczema. Depression, fatigue and a chronic anaemia are seen. There is an increased incidence of inflammatory bowel disease, spondyloarthropathies and pyoderma gangrenosum.

Clinical Features

The characteristic features are deep-seated nodules and abscesses in the axillae, groins and vulva (Figure 14.1). The breasts, inframammary areas and buttocks may be involved with extension on to the thighs in severe cases. Some of the nodules may have an overgranulated appearance and bridged comedones are often seen (Figure 14.2). Squamous cell carcinoma has been reported to occur in severe HS but is more common in males. The perineum is a common site.

A clinical grading system (Hurley stages 1–3) is useful to score disease severity (Table 14.1).

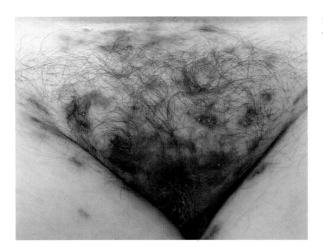

Figure 14.1 Hidradenitis suppurativa – vulval involvement.

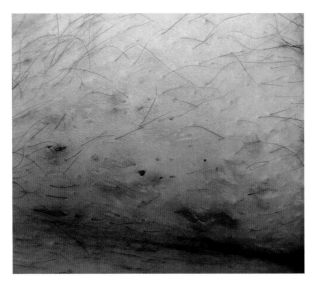

Figure 14.2 Bridged comedones.

Table 14.1 Hurley staging system for hidradenitis supparativa.

Hurley stage	Clinical features
I	Single or multiple nodules or abscesses but without scarring or sinus tracts
II	Recurrent abscesses with single or separate sinus tracts
III	Diffuse involvement with multiple interconnected abscesses

Basic Management

Weight reduction and stopping smoking are very important as general measures. Further management is then based on the stage of the disease.

Medical Management

Stage I Disease

Topical antibiotic treatment such as topical clindamycin 1%, may be sufficient but this needs to be used for at least 12 weeks.

Stage II Disease

Oral treatment is usually required and the first-line treatment is oral antibiotics. Tetracyclines are most commonly used for their anti-inflammatory properties, for example oxytetracycline 500 mg bd or lymecycline 408 mg od or bd. Patients must be counselled to avoid pregnancy while taking these drugs as they can affect the development of the bones and teeth in the foetus.

The combination of clindamycin and rifampicin (both given at 300 mg bd) for 12 weeks has been shown to be helpful. The course can be repeated but long-term treatment is not recommended because of bacterial resistance and side effects. Clindamycin can cause diarrhoea and patients should be warned that rifampicin can colour the urine and tears orange.

Anti-androgens may help some women. Isotretinoin is not generally helpful and as it is severely teratogenic, it is often not suitable to use in young women. Acitretin has been used but again has teratogenic potential.

Stage III Disease

These patients should be referred to a dermatologist as other systemic options may be required. Cyclosporine, azathioprine and biologic therapy such as infliximab or adalimumab may be needed.

Surgery

Lesions frequently recur after simple incision and drainage but more extensive surgery can be helpful in those with severe disease where medical management has failed. A range of techniques from deroofing of tracts and limited excision to extensive excision of all hair-bearing skin with grafting can be used and needs to be tailored to the individual patient.

Laser therapy, photodynamic therapy and radiotherapy have been used with limited effect.

When to Refer

- Hurley stage 2/3.
- Patients requiring surgery.

- Check other sites for disease.
- Treatment can take a long time to take effect and should be continued for 12 weeks in most cases.

Further Reading

Alikhan, A., Lynch, P. J. and Eisen, D. B. (2009) Hidradenitis suppurativa; a comprehensive review. *Journal of the American Academy of Dermatology* **60**(4), 539–561.

Gener, G., Canoui-Poitrine, F., Revuz, J. E. *et al.* (2009) Combination therapy with clindamycin and rifampicin for hidradentitis suppurativa: a series of 116 consecutive patients. *Dermatology* **219**, 148–154.

Hughes, R., Kelly, G., Sweeny, C. *et al.* (2015) The medical and laser management of hidradenitis suppurativa. *American Journal of Clinical Dermatology* **16**(2), 111–123.

Jemec, G. B. (2012) Clinical practice. Hidradenitis suppurativa. *New England Journal of Medicine* **12**, 366(2): 188.

Useful Web Sites for Patient Information

British Association of Dermatologists:
http://www.bad.org.uk/shared/get-file.ashx?id=88&itemtype=document (accessed 14 September 2016)

DermNet:
http://www.dermnetnz.org/acne/hidradenitis-suppurativa.html (accessed 14 September 2016)

Hidradentitis Suppurativa Foundation:
www.hs-foundation.org (accessed 14 September 2016)

Hidradenitis Suppurativa Trust:
www.hstrust.org (accessed 14 September 2016)

International Society for the Study of Vulvovaginal Disease:
http://www.issvd.org/hidradenitis-suppurativa/ (accessed 18 September 2016)

Crohn's Disease

Introduction

Crohn's disease is a chronic granulomatous disease of the gastrointestinal tract. Cutaneous involvement can occur perianally as direct extension of the bowel disease but separate distant lesions can occur and are then termed 'metastatic' – but 'noncontiguous' is probably a better term as there is no malignant link with these lesions. Characteristic vulval lesions can occur with or without gastrointestinal disease.

Epidemiology

Crohn's disease is more common in women and can start in childhood. Extraintestinal manifestations may affect up to 35% of patients and these can affect the skin, eyes, mouth and joints. Cutaneous lesions can include erythema nodosum and pyoderma gangrenosum. Lesions involving the vulva can occur in 20% of those with Crohn's disease and sometimes these can precede the development of gastro-intestinal disease by many years.

Pathophysiology

It is though that activation of T lymphocytes producing the cytokines interleukin-12 and TNF alpha leads to the inflammation seen in Crohn's disease. There may be a genetic predisposition to the disease.

Histological Features

The histological features vary in Crohn's disease. Mild oedema with dilated lymphatics may be the only feature. Noncaseating granulomata with a perivascular distribution are considered characteristic.

Symptoms

Patients with Crohn's disease complain of swelling with pain and discomfort if the skin ulcerates. Ulcers may produce a serous or pus-like discharge. A watery discharge is common from lymphangiectasia if present. Bowel symptoms include abdominal pain, bloody diarrhoea and weight loss.

Clinical Features

The presenting feature of vulval Crohn's disease is often oedema (Figure 14.3). This is usually bilateral and generally affects both the labia majora and minora. The oedema can then become chronic and leads to the development of hypertrophic masses. Lymphangiectasia may be a significant feature in some patients (Figure 14.4). Fissuring and ulceration are common and the fissures have a very

Figure 14.3 Oedema in ano-genital Crohn's disease may be the only feature.

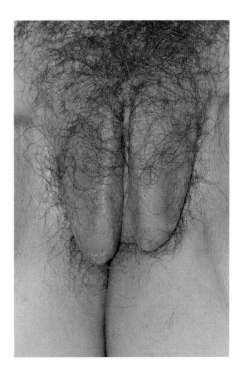

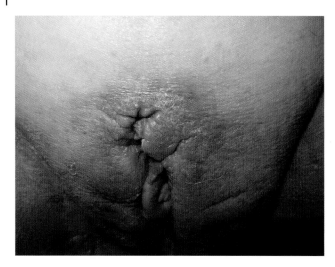

Figure 14.4 Lymphangiectasia are a frequent feature.

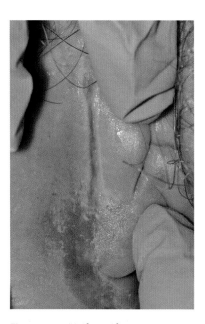

Figure 14.5 'Knife-cut' fissures.

characteristic 'knife-cut' appearance (Figure 14.5). They are often deep and painful affecting the interlabial sulci, inguinal folds and gluteal cleft (Figure 14.6). Similar linear fissures may develop in lower abdominal surgical scars (Figure 14.7).

Some patients have nodules and abscesses with clinical features that overlap with hidradenitis suppurativa.

Figure 14.6 Fissuring in gluteal cleft.

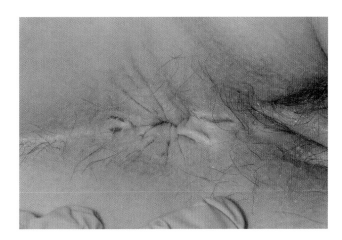

Figure 14.7 Fissuring in abdominal scar.

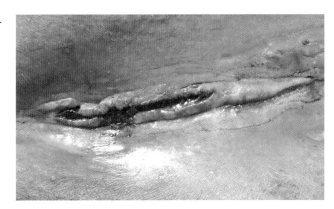

Basic Management

There is no one standard treatment for vulval Crohn's disease. Topical steroids are useful and a potent or ultrapotent preparation can be helpful for the fissures. A prolonged course of antibiotics is first-line treatment but many patients will require systemic immunosuppressive agents or even a biologic agent. It is interesting that the gastrointestinal disease will often respond well to treatment but the cutaneous lesions are more challenging.

When to Refer

- Refer any patient with suspected vulval Crohn's disease as they need specialist management.

Practice Points

- Ask about gastrointestinal symptoms in those with typical vulval features and refer for a gastroenterology opinion.
- Treatment must be individualized and needs a multi-disciplinary approach

Further Reading

Barret, M., de Parades, V., Battitella, M. *et al.* (2013) Crohn's disease of the vulva. *Journal of Crohn's and Colitis* **10**, 9–16.

Laftah, Z., Bailey, C., Zaheri, S. *et al.* (2015) Vulval Crohn's disease: a clinical study of 22 patients. *Journal of Crohn's and Colitis* **9**(4), 318–325.

Useful Web Sites for Patient Information

Crohn's and Colitis Patient Support Group:
https://www.crohnsandcolitis.org.uk (accessed 18 September 2016)
www.ccfa.org (accessed 14 September 2016)

DermnetL
http://dermnetnz.org/site-age-specific/genital-crohn.html (accessed 14 September 2016)

15

Disorders of Pigmentation on the Vulva

Introduction

Pigmentation can be increased or decreased on the vulva as at other sites. Many lesions that look pigmented on the skin are not always due to increased melanin pigmentation, as vascular lesions and keratinocyte proliferation can also look dark. Increased pigmentation may be diffuse or can occur as discrete lesions. The latter will be discussd separately. Causes of diffuse pigmentation are listed in Table 15.1.

Diffuse pigmentation can occur in those with darker skin types as a variation of normal. In pregnancy, there is increased melanogenesis, which gives rise to facial chloasma, the linea nigra on the abdomen (Figure 15.1) and can also cause darkening of the vulva.

Postinflammatory Pigmentation

A degree of hyperpigmentation is common after almost any inflammatory process on the vulva (Figure 15.2) but it most commonly occurs after lichen planus and a fixed drug eruption. It usually fades but may take many months to do so, particularly in darker skinned individuals. The histology shows pigment incontinence and pigmented macrophages in the dermis.

Post-Traumatic Pigmentation

Trauma is sometimes followed by pigmentation. Obstetric and surgical scars may pigment and this often resolves with time.

Acanthosis Nigricans

Acanthosis nigricans is thought to be caused by factors that increase the proliferation of keratinocytes and dermal fibroblasts. Different types of acanthosis nigricans are given in Table 15.2. There is a strong link with hyperinsulinaemia and insulin. Insulin-like growth factors are thought to be the causative factor. There is also an association with malignancy in some cases and substances secreted by the tumour cause the epidermal growth in these patients. The clinical features of the benign and malignant forms are identical. Sweating, moisture and friction are also factors as acanthosis nigricans has a predilection for body folds such as the neck, axillae (Figure 15.3) and inguinal folds.

A Practical Guide to Vulval Disease: Diagnosis and Management, First Edition. Fiona Lewis, Fabrizio Bogliatto and Marc van Beurden.
© 2017 John Wiley & Sons Ltd. Published 2017 by John Wiley & Sons Ltd.

Table 15.1 Causes of diffuse pigmentation.

	Example
Normal variant	Ethnic groups
Genetic	Dowling–Degos disease (reticular pigmented anomaly of the flexures)
Physiological	Pregnancy
Postinflammatory	After lichen planus
Post-traumatic	After obstetric tears
Metabolic	Acanthosis nigricans
Drug induced	Minocycline
Infection	Tinea, erythrasma
Malignancy	Acanthosis nigricans
Idiopathic	Vulval melanosis

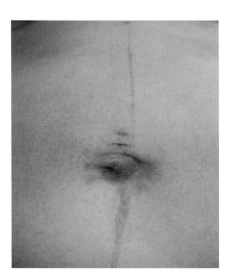

Figure 15.1 Linea nigra.

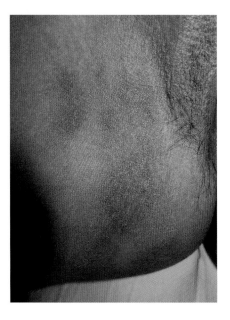

Figure 15.2 Postinflammatory hyperpigmentation after eczema.

Table 15.2 Types of acanthosis nigricans.

Obesity associated	
Endocrine syndromes	Acromegaly
Familial	Autosomal dominant, usually starts in childhood
Drug induced	Nicotinic acid, insulin, steroids
Malignancy	

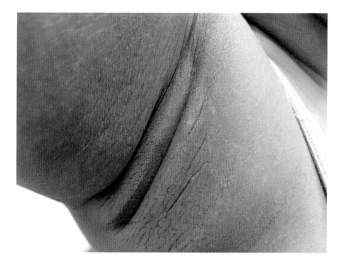

Figure 15.3 Acanthosis nigricans in axilla.

It is estimated that over half of patients who are overweight have a degree of acanthosis nigricans. The malignant form is rare and is often diagnosed at the same time as the malignancy. However, it may occur prior to this diagnosis and in older patients who are not obese with sudden onset of the skin disease; it is important to take a full history and investigate further if necessary. The most commonly associated malignancies are adenocarcinomas of the gastrointestinal tract, especially the stomach (approximately 55% of cases of malignant acanthosis nigricans).

The lesions are thickened and darkened and as they increase in size they form plaques with a velvet surface (Figure 15.4). Skin tags are frequently found on the surface. The inguinal folds and outer labia majora are common sites along with other flexures. The areolae may be involved. The lesions are asymptomatic but the patients may be very troubled by the cosmetic appearance.

There is hyperkeratosis and marked papillomatosis. The darkening of the skin seen clinically is due to the hyperkeratosis. There is no increase in the number of melanocytes or melanin production.

Management

Treatment of any associated hyperinsulinaemia may help, as will weight reduction. Drug-induced acanthosis nigricans can resolve if the causative drug is withdrawn. Surgical excision of any associated tumour has been reported to clear the acanthosis.

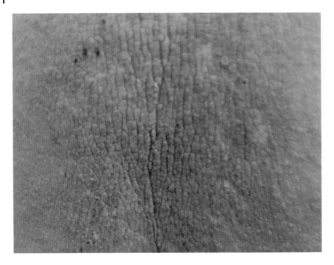

Figure 15.4 Thickened velvety surface seen in acanthosis nigricans.

If persistent, there is no satisfactory treatment. Topical keratolytics such as topical tretinoin 0.05% or 5% salicyclic acid may be helpful in some cases. Dermabrasion and laser therapy may debulk lesions but is not a long-term solution.

Melanosis

Vulval melanosis is common but can often look alarming as it is typically irregular with variable colours from brown to black (Figure 15.5). The main areas affected are the inner aspects of the labia minora and the vestibule. The vagina may be involved and patients sometimes have similar pigmentation in the mouth. A biopsy is mandatory to exclude a melanoma, as the clinical appearances can be very similar (Figure 15.6).

The histology is diagnostic with increased pigmentation of the keratinocytes and melanocytes of the basal layer but no increase in the number of melanocytes (Figure 15.7). Macrophages containing pigment can be seen in the dermis.

It is not thought that melanosis has any potential for progressive change to melanoma but there are no long-term studies. In general, baseline clinical photographs and a biopsy are taken and the patient followed up once a year for a few years to check for any change. In the vast majority of patients there is no alteration in the appearance but a repeat biopsy is recommended in the few patients where there is obvious change.

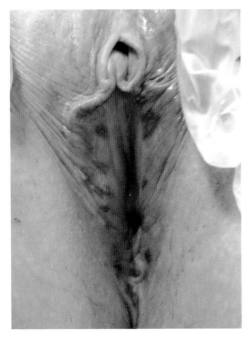

Figure 15.5 Melanosis –irregular pigmentation can be seen in the vestibule.

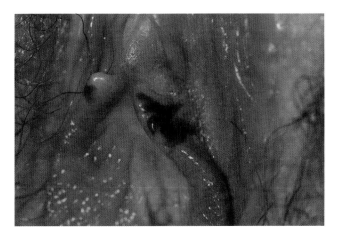

Figure 15.6 Melanosis showing very dark pigmentation.

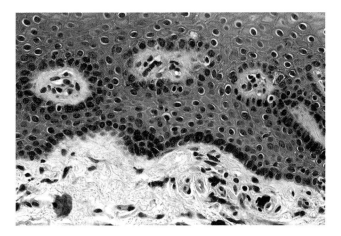

Figure 15.7 Histological features of melanosis – increased melanin and some pigment in the dermis.

Pigmented Lesions

Pigmented lesions may be melanocytic or nonmelanocytic (Table 15.3). Melanocytic lesions are either due to an increase in melanocytes, an increase in melanin production, or pigment incontinence in the dermis.

History and Examination

The history of a pigmented lesion on the vulva may be limited as it is not a visible site and the lesion is usually noticed incidentally as they are rarely symptomatic. Examination of any pigmented lesion should include a detailed description of the lesion itself but it is also important to note the presence of any inflammatory dermatosis or evidence of scarring that may be associated with the pigmentation. It is often very easy for an experienced dermatologist to diagnose a pigmented lesion on keratinized skin by the clinical features alone but this is not so easy on the mucosal

Table 15.3 Pigmented lesions on the vulva.

Melanocytic	Nonmelanocytic	Vascular
Lentigo	Seborrhoeic keratosis	Angiomas
Naevi	Comedones	Angiokeratomas
Atypical genital naevi	Pigmented vulval intraepithelial neoplasia	
Melanoma *in situ*	Pigmented basal cell carcinoma	
Malignant melanoma		

surface of the vulva and histology is often required for an accurate diagnosis. The ABCDE rule for pigmented lesions can be helpful and gives a useful reminder of features to look for:

A – asymmetry
B – border irregular
C – colour – variation in colour
D – diameter >10 mm
E – elevation

Other Techniques

Dermoscopy and confocal microscopy are newer diagnostic techniques that may be useful. However, these require modification of the equipment normally employed at other sites for examination of vulval lesions. It also requires expert interpretation.

Lentigines

These are very common and are seen as smooth dark macules, which are small, measuring just 3–4 mm. Histology shows increased basal layer pigmentation and melanin within dermal macrophages. If numerous, with lesions at other sites, they can be part of some rare syndromes such as LAMB syndrome (lentigines, atrial myxoma, cutaneous myxomas and blue naevi). These patients should be referred for further investigation.

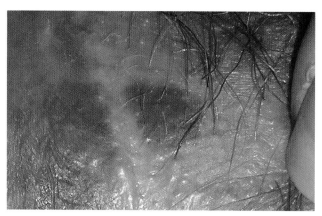

Figure 15.8 Benign mucosal naevus.

Benign Naevi

Vulval naevi are common and may occur in 2.3% of women. Benign naevi may be seen on the labia and these are often single. They are generally flat and macular on mucosal surfaces but with very regular features (Figure 15.8). Compound naevi can occur on the labia majora (Figure 15.9). Histology shows benign nevoid cells with no cytological or architectural atypia. Excision rather than shave excision is recommended, so that the lesion is fully removed and the histological features are not obscured by poor surgical technique.

Atypical Genital Naevi

In patients with a history of atypical naevus syndrome there may be lesions on the vulva as part of this. However, a specific entity of atypical genital naevi can occur in young women (Figure 15.10). These lesions have no increased risk of malignancy but are often misdiagnosed if the pathologist is unaware of the site and the clinical history. The histological features of atypical genital naevi can cause great difficulty in diagnosis and an expert dermatopathological opinion is vital, together with good clinico-pathological correlation, to differentiate these lesions from melanoma.

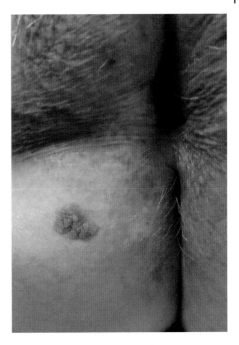

Figure 15.9 Benign compound naevus.

The epidermis is classically hyperplastic. The junctional component of the naevus is nested and commonly involves the adnexal structures as well as the epidermis. The large nests are found along the sides and tips of the rete ridges. The naevoid cells are atypical with this cytological atypia visible in both the junctional and dermal components. Dermal mitoses may be evident.

The interpretation of naevi in patients with lichen sclerosus can also be difficult and requires expert dermatopathological input.

Seborrhoeic Keratoses

These are extremely common and found in most people over the age of 40. The cause is unknown and some patients have multiple lesions. They are frequently found on the vulva, usually on the mons pubis, labia majora or inguinal folds (Figure 15.11). They can mimic pigmented vulval intraepithelial neoplasia and should be biopsied, especially in younger patients.

No treatment is needed but cryotherapy or simple curettage and cautery can be performed if they are troublesome.

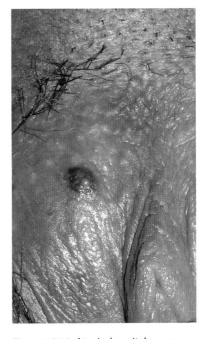

Figure 15.10 Atypical genital naevus.

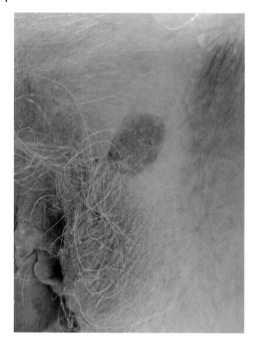

Figure 15.11 Seborrhoeic keratosis.

Pigmented Basal Cell Carcinoma (see Chapter 22)

Vulval basal cell carcinomata are uncommon but when they do occur they are often pigmented. Pigmentation can also occur occasionally in extramammary Paget's disease.

Hypopigmentation

Sometimes there is a loss of pigment after inflammation, more commonly seen in pigmented skin. It can occur after psoriasis or eczematous eruptions.

Vitiligo

Vitiligo is an acquired disorder where there is complete loss of pigment in the skin. The vulva and perianal areas are frequent sites for this and the labia majora and inguinal folds are commonly affected by well defined, symmetrical lesions (Figure 15.12). The texture of the skin is normal and it is totally asymptomatic, with the loss of colour being the only abnormality. The pubic hair may also lose its colour, which is then termed poliosis.

The major differential diagnosis is lichen sclerosus but there is no architectural abnormality in vitiligo and the texture of the skin is normal. However, it is important to remember that vitiligo and lichen sclerosus can coexist, and both disorders are associated with autoimmune disease.

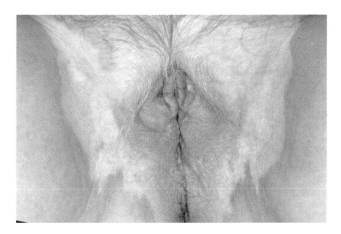

Figure 15.12 Vitiligo (patient also has lichen sclerosus).

No curative treatment exists for vitiligo and treatments that are used at other sites, such as photo-therapy, and psoralen and ultraviolet A radiation (PUVA) are not suitable for the vulva.

When to Refer

- Multiple lentigines where there is the possibility of an associated syndrome.
- Atypical naevi.

Practice Points

- Biopsy any pigmented lesion.
- Expert pathology review and clinic-pathological correlation is very important in the diagnosis of pigmented vulval lesions.

Further Reading

Brenn, T. (2011) Atypical genital naevus. *Archives of Pathology and Laboratory Medicine* **135**, 317–320.

Debarbieux, S., Perrot, J. L., Erfan, N. *et al.* (2014) Reflectance confocal microscopy of mucosal pigmented macules: a review of 56 cases including 10 macular melanomas. *British Journal of Dermatology* **170**, 1276–1284.

Edwards, L. (2010) Pigmented vulvar lesions. *Dermatology and Therapy* **23**, 449–457.

Rock, B., Hood, A. F. and Rock, J. A. (1990) Prospective study of vulvar nevi. *Journal of the American Academy of Dermatology* **22**, 104–106.

Ronger-Savle, S., Julien, V., Duru, G. *et al.* (2011) Features of pigmented vulval lesions on dermoscopy. *British Journal of Dermatology* **164**, 54–61.

Useful Web Sites for Patient Information

DermNet:
http://dermnetnz.org/systemic/acanthosis-nigricans.html (accessed 14 September 2016)

Vitiligo Society:
www.vitiligosociety.org.uk (accessed 14 September 2016)

16

Other Dermatoses

Any dermatological condition has a potential to occur on the genital skin but there are some where involvement at this site is more common (see Table 16.1) and these are discussed here.

Genetic Disorders

Hailey–Hailey Disease (Familial Benign Chronic Pemphigus)

This is a rare blistering disorder inherited as an autosomal dominant trait. The lesions start in the 30s and tend to improve with age but the course is relapsing and remitting. The bullae are intraepidermal and recurrent vesicles and erosions occur in the flexures. The erosions may be crusted, forming plaques with a scaly border (Figure 16.1) and are often initially mistaken for intertrigo or candida infection. The problem is exacerbated by friction, heat and moisture. The outer vulva and inguinal folds are therefore commonly affected.

Histology shows acantholysis in the suprabasal layers of the epidermis. Squamous cell carcinoma has been reported to occur but this is rare.

Management

Simple measures include reducing frictional factors with weight loss being an important part of management. Control of any secondary infection is vital and long-term antibiotics may be required in some patients. Emollients and a moderately potent topical steroid can be helpful in mild disease. Topical tacrolimus has been reported to be of benefit but a case of squamous cell carcinoma developing after treatment has been reported and it should therefore be used with caution. Other options include photodynamic therapy, CO_2 laser, alefacept and botulinum toxin, but the evidence for these treatments is limited.

When to Refer

- If biopsy is required for diagnosis.
- In cases of failure to respond to first-line management or for more severe disease.

Practice Points

- Think of the diagnosis in persistent inflammatory disease of the flexures, not responding to simple measures.
- Ask about family history.

A Practical Guide to Vulval Disease: Diagnosis and Management, First Edition. Fiona Lewis, Fabrizio Bogliatto and Marc van Beurden.
© 2017 John Wiley & Sons Ltd. Published 2017 by John Wiley & Sons Ltd.

Table 16.1 Other dermatoses.

	Example
Genetic disorders	Hailey–Hailey disease
Autoimmune bullous disease	Bullous pemphigoid Pemphigus vulgaris Mucous membrane pemphigoid Bullous dermatosis of childhood
Drug eruptions	Fixed drug eruption Stevens–Johnson syndrome Toxic epidermal necrolysis
Manifestations of underlying disease	Necrolytic migratory erythema Acrodermatitis enteropathica
Inflammatory ulcers	Aphthous ulcers Behcet's disease Lipschtuz ulcers
Others	Graft-versus-host disease Zoon's vulvitis Vulvo-vaginal adenosis Langerhans cell histiocytosis

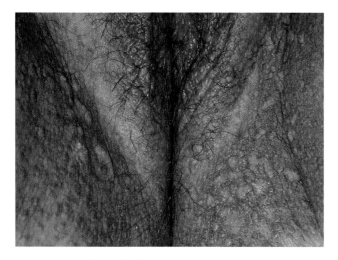

Figure 16.1 Hailey-Hailey disease – pruritic papules on labium majus.

Further Reading

Burge, S. M. (1992) Hailey-Hailey disease: clinical features, response to treatment and prognosis. *British Journal of Dermatology* **126**, 275–282.

Useful Web Site for Patient Information

The Hailey-Hailey disease society:
www.haileyhailey.com (accessed 14 September 2016)

Auto-Immune Bullous Disease

In autoimmune bullous disease (Table 16.2), autoantibodies react against a component of the epidermis or basement membrane to produce a split in the epithelium, which presents as blistering or erosion. The genital area is mainly involved in bullous pemphigoid (BP) and mucous membrane pemphigoid (MMP), where about half of the patients will have some vulval lesions. In linear IgA disease, 80% of children will have vulval involvement and it can present at this site. Pemphigus vulgaris (PV) and epidermolysis bullosa acquisita (EBA) may involve the vulva and vagina less commonly.

The diagnosis is made by taking a skin biopsy and sending for direct immunofluorescence (see Chapter 5) as the patterns seen are specific for each disease. In bullous pemphigoid, mucous membrane pemphigoid and Linear IgA disease, tense blisters are seen (Figure 16.2) as the split in the skin is deep at the level of the dermo-epidermal junction. In pemphigus, blisters are rarely seen as the split is very superficial occurring in the epidermis. Erosions are therefore common.

Table 16.2 Clinical features and immunofluorescence patterns in auto-immune bullous disease.

	Age	Clinical features	Immunofluorescence
Bullous pemphigoid	Elderly	Tense blisters	Linear IgG and C3 at basement membrane (Figure 16.3)
Mucous membrane pemphigoid	Adults, rare in children	Vulval and vaginal lesions with scarring; ocular lesions	Linear IgG at basement membrane
Pemphigus vulgaris	Adults, usually middle aged	Flacid, painful erosions; vaginal disease can cause a discharge	IgG between keratinocytes in epidermis (Figure 16.4)
Linear IgA disease	Children most commonly	Tense blisters, may be clustered in children.	IgA at basement membrane
Epidermolysis bullosa acquisita	Rare, mainly adults	Tense blisters	

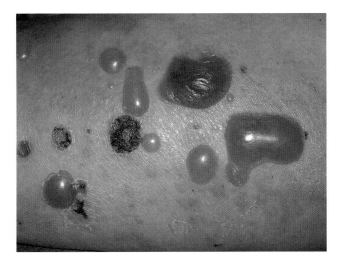

Figure 16.2 Bullous pemphigoid – tense bullae.

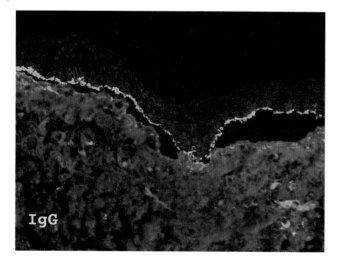

Figure 16.3 Bullous pemphigoid: direct immunofluorescence shows a strong linear deposition of IgG (shown) and C3 both along the basement membrane zone and the roof of the subepidermal blister (courtesy of Dr C. Stefanato)

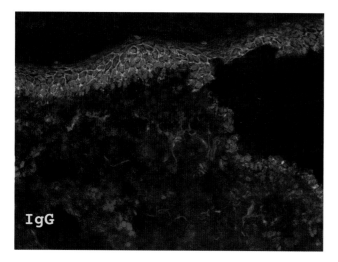

Figure 16.4 Pemphigus: Direct immunofluorescence shows a positive intraepidermal intercellular deposition of IgG (shown) and C3. Please notice the intraepidermal acantholytic blister (courtesy of Dr C Stefanato).

Mucous membrane pemphigoid (cicatrical pemphigoid) is particularly important as the genital lesions lead to scarring (Figure 16.5), which can be difficult to distinguish from lichen planus and lichen sclerosus. The oral lesions are those of a desquamative gingivitis (Figure 16.6). Urethral and vaginal stenosis can occur and perianal lesions lead to pain on defaecation. Ocular involvement can be severe and lead to symblepharon and expert ophthalmological intervention is required in these patients.

In pemphigus vulgaris, vaginal lesions may occur. These can be erosive and scarring is therefore a potential problem. Significant vaginal disease can present with a discharge. The vulval lesions are those of erosions and superficial ulceration (Figure 16.7).

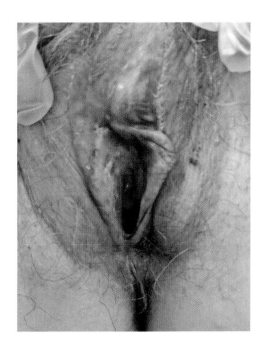

Figure 16.5 Mucous membrane pemphigoid – scarring and erosions.

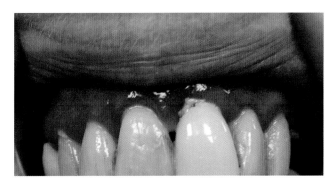

Figure 16.6 Mucous membrane pemphigoid – desquamative gingivitis.

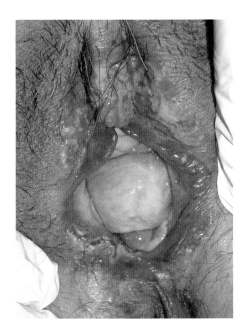

Figure 16.7 Pemphigus vulgaris of the vulva.

- If an autoimmune bullous disease is suspected, refer to a dermatologist as these patients require specialized management with topical and systemic steroids and sometimes immunosuppression.
- Direct immunofluorescence and indirect immunofluorescence is required to make the diagnosis.

Further Reading

Batta, K., Munday, P. E. and Tatnall, F. M. (1999) Pemphigus vulgaris localized to the vagina and presenting as a chronic vaginal discharge. *British Journal of Dermatology* **140**, 945–947.
Marren, P., Wojnarowska, F., Venning, V. *et al.* (1993) Vulvar involvement in auto-immune bullous diseases. *Journal of Reproductive Medicine* **38**, 101–107.

Drug Eruptions

Fixed Drug Eruption

A fixed drug eruption causes the same lesions at the same site every time the drug is ingested and the genital area is one of the preferential sites for this type of drug reaction. It occurs within hours of taking the causative medication and itchy, erythematous lesions develop, which rapidly progress to blisters and erosions. The problem may be intermittent as common agents that cause a fixed drug eruption are analgesics and antibiotics. A very careful history is often required to identify the trigger. Occasionally a challenge test is needed to confirm the diagnosis. The lesions may heal with post-inflammatory hyperpigmentation. The treatment is avoidance as the problem will recur with every exposure to the drug.

Common Drugs Causing a Fixed Drug Eruption
- Nonsteroidal anti-inflammatory drugs.
- Paracetamol.
- Aspirin.
- Antibiotics – tetracyclines and sulphonamides.
- Barbiturates.
- Benzodiazepines.

Further Reading

Fischer, G. (2007) Vulvar fixed drug eruption: a report of 13 cases. *Journal of Reproductive Medicine* **52**, 81–86.
Ozkaya-Bayazit, E. (2003) Specific site involvement in fixed drug eruption. *Journal of the American Academy of Dermatology* **49**, 1003–1007.

Useful Web Site for Patient Information

DermNet:
http://www.dermnetnz.org/reactions/fixed-drug-eruption.html (accessed 14 September 2016)

Stevens–Johnson Syndrome

Erythema multiforme is a cutaneous reactive process either to a drug or infection (most commonly herpes simplex) where typical target lesions are seen. Stevens–Johnson syndrome is a severe form of this where mucosal disease is present in addition to the cutaneous lesions.

Symptoms

The lesions will appear quickly, usually over 24 -48 hours and there may be systemic symptoms with fever and malaise. The oral and vulval lesions are painful. Dysuria may be the presenting feature.

Clinical Features

The lesions are erosive and superficial ulceration may be present (Figure 16.8). These can affect the inner and outer vulva and the vagina can also be involved. Similar lesions can be seen on the oral mucosa and conjunctivae. Secondary bacterial infection can be a problem as the skin barrier is lost. Once the lesions have healed, vulval and vaginal adenosis may develop as postinflammatory complications. If the erosions have been severe, there may be a degree of vaginal stenosis.

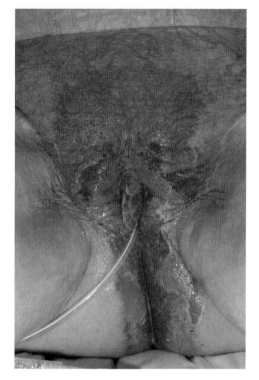

Figure 16.8 Stevens-Johnson syndrome – vulval involvement.

Toxic Epidermal Necrolysis

Toxic epidermal necrolysis (TEN) is a severe, life-threatening condition, most commonly drug induced and characterized by widespread total loss of the epidermis including mucosal epithelium.

Symptoms

Symptoms may start in the flexural areas and the first lesions may be on the vulva. The patient is systemically unwell and cutaneous pain is characteristic.

Clinical Features

Initially, the skin becomes erythematous and Nikolsky's sign is positive (where gentle touch on the skin causes the epidermis to lift off). This is followed by rapid epidermal loss affecting large areas of the skin and mucosa (Figure 16.9). The vulva and vagina are commonly involved. Vaginal stenosis is more common in TEN than in Stevens–Johnson syndrome.

Basic Management

Patients with TEN and Stevens–Johnson syndrome require specialized management and should be urgently transferred to dedicated units for expert nursing and medical care. National protocols and guidelines are available.

The genital lesions are treated with emollients and potent topical steroids. It is important to treat any vaginal involvement as vaginal stenosis can occur rapidly with erosive change. The steroid foam preparations, for example hydrocortisone acetate can be used in the vagina and are applied daily until re-epithelialization occurs.

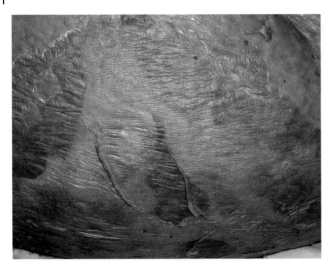

Figure 16.9 Toxic epidermal necrolysis – full thickness epidermal loss.

If vaginal stenosis has occurred, then laser or surgical release of adhesions can be used with post-operative topical steroid application. Laser treatment has also been used for adenosis.

Further Reading

Bonafe, J. I., Thibaut, I. and Hoff, J. (1990) Introital adenosis associated with Stevens-Johnson syndrome. *Clinical and Experimental Dermatology* **15**, 356–357.

Emberger, M., Lanschnetzer, C. M., Laimer, M. *et al.* (2006) Vaginal adenosis induced by Stevens-Johnson syndrome. *Journal of the European Academy of Dermatology and Venereology* **20**, 896–898.

Fromowitz, J. S., Ramos-Caro, F. A. and Flowers, F. P. (2007) Practical guidelines for the management of toxic epidermal necrolysis and Stevens-Johnson syndrome. *International Journal of Dermatology* **46**, 1092–1094.

Meneux, E., Paniel, B. J., Pouget, F. *et al.* (1997) Vulvovaginal sequelae in toxic epidermal necrolysis. *Journal of Reproductive Medicine* **42**, 153–156.

Noel, J. C., Buxant, F., Fayt, I. *et al.* (2005) Vulval adenosis associated with toxic epidermal necrolysis. *British Journal of Dermatology* **153**, 457–458.

Useful Web Site for Patient Information

DermNet:
http://www.dermnetnz.org/reactions/sjs-ten.html (accessed 14 September 2016)

Manifestations of Underlying Disease

Necrolytic Migratory Erythema

This dermatosis is usually related to the glucagonoma syndrome but it is not known how the cutaneous lesions are caused. It does not occur in other conditions where the glucagon levels are raised, so glucagon itself is unlikely to be the cause of the eruption.

Symptoms

The lesions are itchy and then develop into erosions, which dry, crust and then recur in cycles. Moisture and friction can cause new areas to develop.

Clinical Features

The outer labia majora, perineum and perianal skin is involved, with extension into the inguinal folds, thighs and onto the mons pubis and lower abdomen. The lesions are erythematous and often crusted. They spread out to produce annular areas, which can relapse and remit in a cyclical pattern. Postinflammatory hyperpigmentation can last for several weeks afterwards. If associated with a glucagonoma, the eruption rapidly resolves when the glucagonoma is excised.

Basic Management

A skin biopsy will show characteristic features where the keratinocytes are vacuolated and pale. They become necrotic, which leads to intraepidermal clefting and subcorneal pustules. The patient must be referred to an endocrinologist for further investigation and management. A combined potent topical steroid / antibiotic preparation is helpful symptomatically.

Further Reading

Mullans, E. A. and Cohen, P. R. (1998) Iatrogenic necrolytic migratory erythema: a case report and review of nonglucagonoma-associated necrolytic migratory erythema. *Journal of the American Academy of Dermatology* **38**, 866–873.

Nakashima, H., Komina, M., Sasaki, K. *et al.* (2006) Necrolytic migratory erythema without glucagonoma in a patient with short bowel syndrome. *Journal of Dermatology* **33**, 557–562.

Van Beek, A. P., de Haas, E. R., van Vloten, W. A. *et al.* (2004) The glucagonoma syndrome and necrolytic migratory erythema: a clinical review. *European Journal of Endocrinology* **151**, 531–537.

Acrodermatitis Enteropathica

Acrodermatitis enteropathica is a characteristic eruption caused by zinc deficiency. It may be an autosomal recessively inherited disorder but it is more commonly acquired in premature babies or those with malbsorption due to Crohn's disease or other causes. Acrodermatitis enteropathica classically occurs in the first few weeks of life or soon after breastfeeding stops. It can occur in those who are breastfed if the levels of zinc in breast milk are low.

Clinical Features

Bright red lesions, which are often scaly and crusted, mimicking eczema, are seen on the vulva and perineum. They are also found around the mouth. In infants, there is often failure to thrive and a history of diarrhoea. Secondary infection is very common.

Basic Management

The diagnosis is made by measuring the zinc level but if there is a strong suspicion of the diagnosis, it is reasonable to treat empirically with zinc supplements (zinc sulphate or gluconate 1-3 mg/kg/day) while awaiting the result. The lesions rapidly resolve with zinc supplementation.

Practice Point

- Consider acrodermatitis enteropathica if 'eczema' does not respond to treatment, especially in high risk groups such as premature infants and adults with malabsorption.

Further Reading

Bronson, D. M., Barsky, R. and Barsky, S. (1983) Acrodermatitis enteropathica. Recognition at long last during a recurrence in pregnancy. *Journal of the American Academy of Dermatology* **9**, 140–144.

Maverakis, E., Fung, M. A., Lynch, P. J. *et al.* (2007) Acrodermatitis enteropathica and an overview of zinc metabolism. *Journal of the American Academy of Dermatology* **56**, 116–124.

Perafan-Riveros, C., Franca, L. F., Alves, A. C. and Sanches, J. A. Jr. (2002) Acrodermatitis enteropathica: case report and review of the literature. *Pediatric Dermatology* **19**, 426–431.

Inflammatory Ulcers

Aphthous Ulcers

Aphthous ulcers are recurrent, small ulcers that affect the oral mucosa frequently but the vulva may also be involved, either at the same time or separately. They usually start in childhood and there may be a family history of similar lesions.

Clinical Features

The onset is often sudden with small, painful ulcers, measuring about 1–3 mm on the inner aspects of the labia majora and minora. There is a sloughy base surrounded by a red rim of inflammation (Figure 16.10). Recurrence in the premenstrual period is reported by some women. In some patients, the lesions may be much larger and take longer to resolve. These are commonly called giant or major aphthae.

Management

A mild to moderate topical steroid preparation can aid healing and 5% lidocaine ointment is helpful for local pain relief. There may be a relationship with low levels of B_{12} or folate in these patients and if low, this should be replaced with oral supplements.

Practice Point

- Differentiate the lesions from herpes simplex as they will recur in different areas and vesicles are not seen.

Behcet's Syndrome

Behcet's syndrome is a multisystem inflammatory disorder of unknown aetiology but immune dysregulation triggers an inflammatory reaction in genetically predisposed individuals. It is more common in Mediterranean countries along the silk route. There is no specific diagnostic test and the diagnosis is made clinically based on diagnostic criteria (Table 16.3). The patient must have recurrent oral ulcers plus at least two minor criteria.

Figure 16.10 Healing aphthous ulcer lower right labium majus.

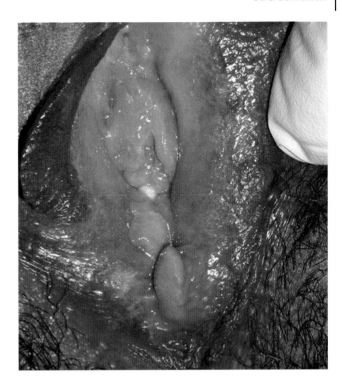

Table 16.3 Diagnostic criteria for Behcet's syndrome.

Major criteria	Minor criteria
Recurrent oral ulcers occurring at least three times in 12 months	Genital ulcers
	Skin lesions – folliculitis, erythema nodosum, superficial thrombophlebitis
	Eye symptoms – iritis, uveitis, retinal vasculitis
	Pathergy – pustule formation at site of minor injury, e.g. phlebotomy site
	Arthritis/arthralgia
	Neurological symptoms

The genital ulcers are typically large and deep and heal with scarring (Figure 16.11), which can distinguish them from aphthous ulcers. They can be treated with a topical steroid and, if painful, a topical local anaesthetic can be useful, particularly for micturition.

Treatment is aimed at suppressing the inflammation and to prevent end-organ damage. Patients should be managed in multidisciplinary clinics with access to a range of specialists who may be required for the varying manifestations.

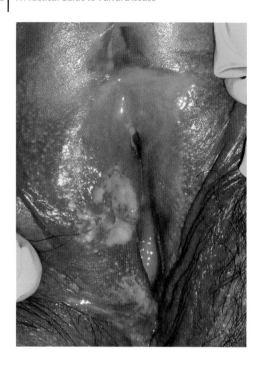

Figure 16.11 Behcet's disease – deeper scarring ulcers.

Further Reading

Ideguchi, H., Suda, A., Takeno, M. *et al.* (2011) Behcet disease: evolution of clinical manifestations. *Medicine* **90**, 125–132.

International Study Group for Behcet's Disease Criteria for diagnosis of Behcet's disease (1990). *Lancet* **335**, 1078–1080.

Useful Resources

The Behcet's Society:
www.behcets.org.uk (accessed 14 September 2016)

Lipschutz Ulceration

Lipschtuz ulcers (ulcus vulvae acutum), first described by Lipschutz in 1913, are acute vulval ulcers occurring typically in teenagers and young adults. They develop quickly over about 24–48 hours and are usually a reactive process to infection. They have been most commonly reported after Epstein–Barr infection but other infections including typhoid, paratyphoid and mumps have also been linked.

Clinical Features

The ulcers are painful and develop rapidly. There may be a history of preceding systemic features or a sore throat. The ulcers can become large, involving almost the whole of the inner labia majora (Figure 16.12). They are often bilateral, giving rise to the so-called 'kissing ulcers'. The base is sloughy but secondary infection is not very common. They heal spontaneously over 10 days to 2 weeks and do not generally recur.

Basic Management

The diagnosis is clinical and it is important to make this early to avoid unnecessary surgical intervention with debridement or excision. Viral serology can be done to confirm any associated infection but may be negative.

If the ulcers are small, a topical steroid alone may be sufficient for treatment. For larger lesions, a short course of oral prednisolone, for example 15–20 mg/day for 10 days, is helpful to aid resolution. Simple oral analgesics and 5% lidocaine ointment can help to relieve the symptoms, as micturition is often painful.

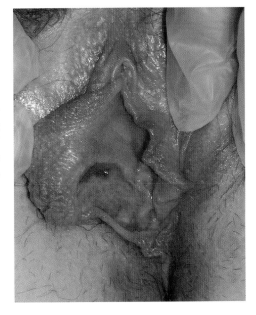

Figure 16.12 Lipschutz ulcer.

Further Reading

Barnes, C. J., Alio, A. B., Cunningham, B. B. *et al.* (2007) Epstein–Barr virus associated genital ulcers: an under-recognised disorder. *Paediatric Dermatology* **24**, 130.

Chanal, J., Carlotti, A., Lande, H. *et al.* (2010) Lipschutz gential ulceration associated with mumps. *Dermatology* **221**, 292–295.

Halvorsen, J. A., Brevig, T., Aas, T. *et al.* (2006) Genital ulcers as initial manifestation of Epstein–Barr virus infection: two new cases and review of the literature. *Acta Dermato-Venereologica* **86**, 439–442.

Lipschutz, B. (1913) Über eine eigenartige Geschwüursform des weiblichen Genitales (ulcus vulvae acutum). *Archives of Dermatology Syphilis (Berlin)* **114**, 363–396.

Portnoy, J., Arontheim, G. A., Ghibu, F. *et al.* (1984) Recovery of Epstein–Barr virus from genital ulcers. *New England Journal of Medicine* **311**, 966–968.

Others

Graft-Versus-Host Disease

Graft-versus-host disease (GVHD) occurs after allogeneic stem cell transplant, and is due to the donor cells reacting against host tissue. It can affect the skin and mucous membranes in two main clinical patterns – the lichenoid and sclerodermoid types. The female genital tract can be involved in almost half the patients and the condition can be severe but is often not recognized and treated early as the management of serious pulmonary and gastrointestinal complications takes priority.

Erythema and erosions are seen in the vulva and vagina (Figure 16.13) and the clinical appearances are often completely indistinguishable from those seen in erosive lichen planus. Erosions rapidly lead to scarring and stenosis and may patients present at this stage. Ultrapotent topical steroids can be used to treat the vulva. Hydrocortisone acetate foam inserted intravaginally with the use of regular dilators to maintain patency are needed for the vaginal disease. If stenosis has occurred then expert surgical intervention is required with careful post-operative care in the same way as that for erosive lichen planus (see Chapter 13). Patients may require systemic immune suppressions as recommended by the haematologists and extracorporeal photophoresis is available in a few specialized centres.

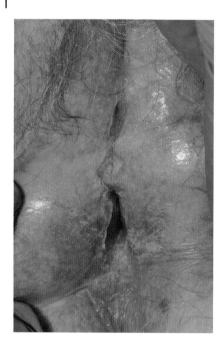

Figure 16.13 Genital graft-versus-host disease – appearances may be indistinguishable from erosive lichen planus.

Further Reading

Ciavattini, A. and Clements, N. (2015) Female genital tract chronic graft versus host disease: review of the literature. *Anticancer Research* **35**, 13–17.

Dignan, F., Clark, A., Amrolia, P. *et al.* (2012) Diagnosis and management of acute graft-versus-host disease. *British Journal of Haematology* **158**, 30–45.

Hirsch, P., Leclerc, M., Rybojad, M. *et al.* (2012) Female genital chronic graft-versus-host disease: importance of early diagnosis to avoid severe complications. *Transplantation* **93**, 1265–1269.

Zantomio, D., Grigg, A. P., MacGregor, L. *et al.* (2006) Female genital tract graft versus host disease: incidence, risk factors and recommendations for management. *Bone Marrow Transplant* **38**, 567–572.

Zoon's Vulvitis (Plasma Cell Vulvitis)

Although Zoon's balanitis is a well defined entity, true Zoon's vulvitis is less common and many of the reports have significant overlap with lichen planus. It may represent a reaction pattern to another inflammatory process. Plasma cells are a very common finding in inflammatory conditions in the vestibule and so the condition may be labelled as plasma cell vulvitis, especially if the biopsy is taken from the vestibular area.

Histology

The histological features that should be present to diagnose Zoon's vulvitis are a thinned epidermis with no granular cell layer, spongiosis and a dense band of dermal inflammation containing many plasma cells. The keratinocytes are often lozenge or diamond shaped.

Symptoms

Patients may complain of itching or discomfort but it may be asymptomatic and the changes may be noticed at routine examination.

Clinical Features

The labia minora and vestibule are most commonly affected and erythematous glazed patches with a typical 'beefy-red' or brown appearance, due to deposition of haemosiderin, are seen (Figure 16.14). Purpuric lesions are sometimes seen. This is sometimes termed chronic vulval purpura.

Basic Management

Emollients and a potent topical steroid if there are any features of associated lichen planus. Misoprostol has been reported to be of use but tacrolimus does not seem to be beneficial.

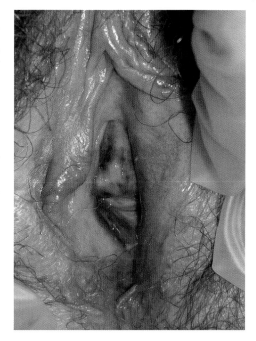

Figure 16.14 Zoon's vulvitis.

Further Reading

Gunter, J. and Golitz, L. (2005) Topical misoprostol therapy for plasma cell vulvitis: a case series. *Journal of Lower Genital Tract Disorders* **9**, 176–180.

Li, Q., Leopold, K. and Carlson, J. A. (2003) Chronic vulvar purpura: persistent pigmented purpuric dermatitis (lichen aureus) of the vulva or plasma cell (Zoon's) vulvitis? *Journal of Cutaneous Pathology* **30**, 572–576.

Scurry, J., Dennerstein, G. and Brennan, J. (1993) Vulvitis corcumscripta. A clinico-pathological entity? *Journal of Reproductive Medicine* **38**, 14–18.

Virgili, A., Mantovani, L., Lauriola, M. M. *et al.* (2008) Tacrolimus 0.1% ointment: is it really effective in plasma cell vulvitis? *Dermatology* **216**, 243–246.

Vulvovaginal Adenosis

Vulvovaginal adenosis describes metaplastic cervical or endometrial epithelium in the vulva and vagina. The aetiology is unknown but one theory is that it may develop from remnants of paramesonephric tissue.

It may occur as a consequence of severe inflammatory erosive disease such as toxic epidermal necrolysis or Stevens–Johnson syndrome but also follows the prolonged use of the oral contraceptive pill. Previously, when diethyl stilboestrol was sometimes taken during pregnancy, adenosis in the upper vagina was seen after *in utero* exposure, and was associated with vaginal adenocarcinoma.

The lesions are erythematous and may be uncomfortable. Itching is not generally described. Laser treatment has been reported to be useful.

Further Reading

Emberger, M., Lanschnetzer, C. M., Laimer, M. *et al.* (2006) Vaginal adenosis induced by Stevens–Johnson syndrome. *Journal of the European Academy of Dermatology and Venereology* **20**, 896–898.

Yaghsezian, H., Palazzo, J. P., Finkel, G. C. *et al.* (1992) Primary vaginal adenocarcinoma of the intestinal type associated with adenosis. *Gynecologic Oncology* **45**, 62–65.

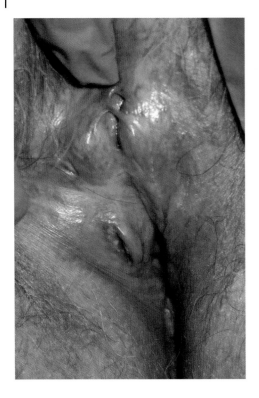

Figure 16.15 Langerhans cell histiocytosis of the vulva.

Langerhans Cell Histiocytosis

This condition is an abnormal proliferation of tumour cells that resemble normal Langerhans cells. The histological features are the presence of large cells with a 'coffee-bean' nucleus and Langerhans cells expressing CD1a, S100 and langerin (CD207), which is a specific marker. On electron microscopy, Birkbeck granules are seen and these are considered pathognomonic.

The vulva can be involved with papules, plaques and ulcerated lesions (Figure 16.15). Patients require investigation to exclude disease at other sites because the lungs, hypothalamic-pituitary axis, bones and reticulo-endothelial system may all be involved. Localized radiotherapy, surgery and chemotherapy are used in management.

Further Reading

Jiang, W., Li, L., He, Y. M. and Yang, K. X. (2012) Langerhans cell histiocytosis of the female genital tract: a literature review with additional three case studies in China. *Archives of Gynecology and Obstetrics* **285**, 99–103.

17

Vulval Infection – Sexually Transmitted

Normal Flora

Most studies of the microbiology of the lower genital tract relate to the vaginal flora. The micro-environment at this site is a self-regulating, self-cleaning, resilient yet delicate ecosystem. There is not so much information about the vulva. The vulva of the newborn child is sterile but after the first 24 hours of life it gradually acquires, from the skin, vagina and intestine, a rich varied flora of non-pathogenic organisms. The vulval flora is mainly composed of Gram-positive bacteria such as Staphylococcus species including *S. aureus, S. epidermidis, S. saprophyticus* and *S. pyogenes.* The close proximity to the vagina, the urethra, and the anus, may result in contamination with the flora typical for those sites, such as lactobacilli, candida species, Group B Streptococcus, and *Gardnerella vaginalis.* In certain situations, (a moist environment, antibiotic medication, radiotherapy and chemotherapy, immunosuppression) these microorganisms may increase their pathogenicity, causing a vulvitis.

Infections affecting the vulva and vagina may be sexually or nonsexually transmitted. The main sexually transmitted infections (STIs) are listed in Table 17.1 by their causative organisms. More than one sexually transmitted infection may occur in the same patient and therefore any patient with a suspected or confirmed STI must be referred to a genito-urinary clinic for full screening, contact tracing and expert management.

Trichomoniasis

Trichomoniasis is a common sexually transmitted infection with over 3 million people infected in the United States each year. It can be associated with prematurity and low birth weight if it occurs during pregnancy. There is also a link with HIV infection and trichomoniasis may increase the risk of transmission of HIV.

Pathophysiology

The causative organism is the protozoan *Trichomonas vaginalis.* It is found in the vagina but 90% of infected women have urethral infection.

A Practical Guide to Vulval Disease: Diagnosis and Management, First Edition. Fiona Lewis, Fabrizio Bogliatto and Marc van Beurden.
© 2017 John Wiley & Sons Ltd. Published 2017 by John Wiley & Sons Ltd.

Table 17.1 Major sexually transmitted infections.

Protozoa	Trichomoniasis
Bacteria	Chlamydia
	Lymphogranuloma venereum
	Gonorrhoea
	Syphilis
	Chancroid
	Donovanosis
Viruses	Herpes simplex infection
	Human papilloma virus infection
	Molluscum contagiosum
Parasites	Scabies
	Pubic lice

Clinical Features

The main symptom is a vaginal discharge which may be malodorous. Dysuria and vulval pruritus are also common. However, up to 50% of patients do not report any symptoms. The discharge is typically foamy but can vary in type and a 'strawberry' like appearance is seen on the cervix. Vestibular erythema and posterior vulvitis is seen secondary to the vaginal discharge.

Diagnosis

The diagnosis can be made by direct microscopy of a wet preparation as the motile organisms are easily seen. The infection can then be confirmed on culture. Several nucleic acid amplification tests are now used, and these are regarded as the most sensitive tests.

Basic Management

The treatment is a single dose of 2 g of metronidazole. The patient should be referred to a genito-urinary clinic for contact tracing and screening for other STIs.

Further Reading

Forna, F. and Gulmezoglu, A. M. (2003) Interventions for treating trichomoniasis in women. *Cochrane Database of Systematic Reviews* **2** (Art. No.: CD000218).

Sherrard, J., Ison, C., Moody, J. *et al.* (2014) UK National Guideline on the management of trichomas vaginalis 2014. *International Journal of STD and AIDS* **25**, 541–549.

Useful Web Site for Patient Information

British Association for Sexual Health and HIV:

http://www.bashh.org/documents/TV%20PIL%20Screen%20-%20Edit.pdf (accessed 14 September 2016)

http://www.bashh.org/documents/TV_2014%20IJSTDA.pdf (accessed 14 September 2016).

CDC Guidelines on Treatment:
http://www.cdc.gov/std/tg2015/trichomoniasis.htm (accessed 14 September 2016).
http://www.cdc.gov/std/trichomonas/stdfact-trichomoniasis.htm (accessed 14 September 2016)

Chlamydia

Chlamydia trachomatis is a bacterium with two distinct biovars that cause genital disease (D-K) and eye disease (A-C) respectively. Genital chlamydia is one of the most common sexually transmitted infections in the young, affecting up to 10% of sexually active women under the age of 24. Rectal and pharyngeal infections may also occur but are less common.

Clinical Features

The infection is asymptomatic in 70% of infected females. A vaginal discharge or bleeding may occur with or without abdominal pain or dysuria. If untreated, 40% of patients may then go on to develop pelvic inflammatory disease. Clinical examination is often normal. A purulent discharge and contact bleeding in the vagina may be seen.

Diagnosis

Cervical or vulvo-vaginal swabs or urine samples are taken and nucleic acid amplification techniques are used to test for the organism.

Treatment

The recommended treatment is 1 g of azithromycin.

Further Reading

Malhotra, M., Sood, S., Mukherjee, A. *et al.* (2013) Genital chlamydia trachomatis: an update. *Indian Journal of Medical Research* **138**, 303–316.

Useful Web Site for Patient Information

CDC guidelines on treatment:
http://www.cdc.gov/std/tg2015/chlamydia.htm (accessed 14 September 2016)

Lymphogranuloma Venereum

Lymphogranuloma venereum (LGV) is a sexually transmitted infection where the causative organism is a serovar of *Chlamydia trachomatis,* most commonly L2. The incidence has been increasing, especially among HIV-positive men who have sex with men.

Clinical Features

In women, the initial lesion is a painless, shallow erosion on the vulva or vaginal wall. Painful regional lymphadenopathy is common and buboes may develop. If the disease spreads, destructive lesions, fistulae, chronic granulomatous inflammation and oedema may ensue (Figure 17.1).

Diagnosis

Nucleic acid amplification tests are now routinely used.

Treatment

Doxycycline 100 mg bd for 21 days is used as a first-line treatment. Other antibiotics include minocycline or erythromycin.

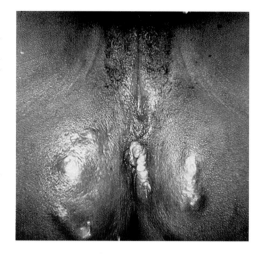

Figure 17.1 Lymphogranuloma venereum: sinuses.

Further Reading

White, J., O'Farrell, N. and Daniels, D. (2013) UK national guideline for the management of lymphogranuloma venereum. *International Journal of STI and AIDS* **24**, 593–601.

Useful Web Site for Patient Information

CDC 2015 guidance:
http://www.cdc.gov/std/tg2015/lgv.htm (accessed 14 September 2016)

Gonorrhoea

The causative organism of gonorrhoea is Neisseria *gonorrhoea*, a Gram-negative diplococcus. Transmission is via direct contact with infected secretions and common sites of infection are the cervix, urethra, rectum and pharynx.

Clinical Features

About half of the females infected are asymptomatic. A vaginal discharge, dysuria and abdominal pain may occur. Examination may be normal but a purulent discharge is sometimes visible. Infection may spread to cause Bartholin's gland enlargement and even abscess formation. Further spread can lead to pelvic inflammatory disease and even disseminated infection with arthritis and cutaneous lesions.

Diagnosis

Nucleic acid amplification tests are increasingly used as the most sensitive test. The organisms can be seen on direct microscopy of a discharge and then cultured.

Treatment

A cephalosporin is the treatment of choice but other regimens are published and expert advice should be sought as there are problems with antibiotic resistance.

Further Reading

Bignell, C. and Fitzgerald, M. (2011) UK national guidelines for the management of gonorrhoea in adults 2011. *International Journal of STD and AIDS* **22**, 541–547.

Useful Web Sites for Patient Information

British Association for Sexual Health and HIV:
http://www.bashh.org/documents/3920.pdf (accessed 14 September 2016).

CDC guidelines and patient information:
http://www.cdc.gov/std/gonorrhea/ (accessed 14 September 2016)

Syphilis

Syphilis is due to infection with the spirochaete *Treponema pallidum.* It presents in one of four different stages: primary, secondary, latent, and tertiary. Primary syphilis is typically acquired by direct sexual contact with an infectious lesion. There has been rise in the number of cases of syphilis in Europe and the United States since the 1990s.

Pathophysiology

The causative organism enters via small breaks in the mucosa or skin. After 3 to 90 days from the initial exposure (average 21 days) a skin lesion appears at the point of contact. This chancre contains millions of spirochaetes. These spread via the bloodstream to other organs at this stage and transplacental transmission is also common at this point. This may give rise to systemic symptoms associated with secondary syphilis.

Clinical Features

Lesions occur on the vulva in only 2–7% of cases as the most common location in women is the cervix (44%). In 80% of cases, inguinal lymph node enlargement is present. The lesion may persist for 3 to 6 weeks without treatment. This is described in many patients as a single, firm, painless, non-itchy ulcer (Figure 17.2) but they may be painful in 30%.

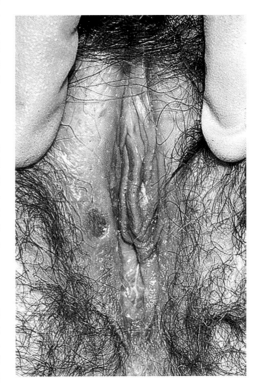

Figure 17.2 Primary chancre of syphilis on right inner labium majus.

They usually have a clean base and sharp borders measuring between 0.3 and 3.0 cm in size. The lesion, however, may take on almost any form. In the classic form, it evolves from a macule to a papule and finally to an erosion or ulcer. Occasionally, multiple lesions may be present.

Secondary syphilis occurs approximately 4 to 10 weeks after the primary infection. While secondary disease is known for the many different manifestations (it has been termed the 'great mimicker'), symptoms most commonly involve the skin. It presents as a symmetrical, reddish-pink, non-itchy rash on the trunk and extremities, including the palms and soles. Oral ulceration ('snail track' ulcers) and condylomata lata occur at this stage. The condylomata lata are warty lesions on the vulva and perianal area.

The acute symptoms usually resolve after 3 to 6 weeks; however, about 25% of people may present with a recurrence of secondary symptoms. Many people who present with secondary syphilis (40–85% of women, 20–65% of men) do not report previously primary syphilis.

Latent syphilis is defined as having serologic proof of infection without symptoms of disease. It usually presents less than 1 year after secondary syphilis or later. Late latent syphilis is asymptomatic and not as contagious as early latent syphilis.

Tertiary syphilis may occur approximately 3 to 15 years after the initial infection and may be divided into three different forms: gummatous syphilis (15%); late neurosyphilis (6.5%); and cardiovascular syphilis (10%). Without treatment, a third of infected people develop tertiary disease. People with tertiary syphilis are not infectious.

Treatment

Treatment of early syphilis is a single dose of intramuscular benzathine penicillin G. Doxycycline and tetracycline are alternative choices for those allergic to penicillin. It is recommended that treated patients avoid sexual intercourse until the sores are healed. Expert advice must be taken for pregnant patients for the management of potential congenital syphilis.

Further Reading

Clement, M. E., Okeke, N. L. and Hicks, C. B. (2014) Treatment of syphilis; a systematic review. *Journal of the American Medical Association* **312**, 1905–1917.

Useful Web Site for Patient Information

CDC 2015 guidance on syphilis:
http://www.cdc.gov/std/syphilis/ (accessed 14 September 2016)

Chancroid

Chancroid was a major cause of genital ulceration but the incidence has dropped significantly in recent years.

Pathophysiology

The causative organism of chancroid is *Haemophilus ducreyi*, a Gram-negative anaerobic bacillus.

Clinical Features

The pathogen infects its host by way of breaks in the skin or epidermis. The lesion starts as an erythematous papule that breaks down into a painful bleeding ulcer with a necrotic base and ragged edge. These occur on the labia but also in the vagina and cervix. Lymphadenopathy can occur and may be associated with the development of a bubo.

Treatment

It is best treated with a macrolide like azithromycin and a third-generation cephalosporin like ceftriaxone.

Further Reading

O'Farrell, N. and Lazaro, N. (2014) UK national guidelines for the management of chancroid 2014. *International Journal of STI and AIDS* **25**, 975–983.

Useful Web Sites for Patient Information

British Association for Sexual Health and HIV:
http://www.bashh.org/documents/Chancroid%20PIL%20Screen%20-%20Edit.pdf (accessed 14 September 2016)

2015 CDC guidelines on sexually transmitted disease
http://www.cdc.gov/std/tg2015/chancroid.htm (accessed 14 September 2016)

Donovanosis (Granuloma Inguinale)

Donovanosis is rare outside the endemic areas of Papua New Guinea, areas of India, Africa and South America. It is caused by *Klebsiella granulomatis.*

Clinical Features

A papule develops at the site of inoculation, which develops into painless ulcers. These can be large and irregular. The inguinal lymph nodes can form abscesses and ulcerate. Lymphoedema and malignancy are complications.

Diagnosis

Donovan bodies (Gram-negative capsulated bodies in the histiocytes) are seen on histological examination with Giemsa or Warthin Starry stains.

Treatment

There are a few antibiotic regimes used including cotrimaoxazole, azithromycin and doxycycline, usually given for 3 weeks until all lesions have resolved.

Further Reading

O'Farrell, N., Moi, H. and the IUSTI/WHO European STD Guidelines Editorial Board (2010) European guideline for the management of donovanosis 2010. *International Journal of STD and AIDS* **21**, 609–610.

Useful Web Site for Patient Information

CDC guidance on donovanosis:
http://www.cdc.gov/std/tg2015/donovanosis.htm (accessed 14 September 2016)

Herpes Simplex Infection

Vulval herpes is a genital infection caused by the herpes simplex virus (HSV) types 1 and 2. It is one of the major causes of consultation in genito-urinary clinics. Its prevalence is estimated to be 20 per 100 adults. Most patients who transmit genital herpes to a sexual partner or at delivery do not have a history of lesions at the time of transmission, suggesting that asymptomatic viral shedding or unrecognized lesions are responsible in most cases of infection.

Incidence

Herpes simplex infection is the most common human infection. The frequency of HSV 1 and 2 infection has been measured by testing various populations for the presence of antibodies, as both the virus and the immune response persist after infection. Worldwide, 90% of people have evidence of infection with one or both viruses.

Pathophysiology

The principal mode of transmission is direct contact with infected secretions. After exposure to HSV, primary infection may occur followed by spontaneous regression, normally in 15–17 days. A quarter of patients are asymptomatic. After the primary infection, the virus remains latent in the dorsal root nerve ganglia nearest to the original site of infection. Reactivation causes viral shedding and outbreaks on the genital area and other sites. The signs and symptoms of genital herpes caused by HSV-1 or HSV-2 are indistinguishable. The periods of asymptomatic viral shedding and recurrence rates are unpredictable.

Clinical Features

The symptoms of genital herpes infection are described as pain, burning and dysuria. Some patients may experience systemic symptoms and fever but others have no symptoms or such mild symptoms that an infection is not suspected. The first episode of herpes (primary infection) can cause one or more very painful lesions to erupt on the skin whereas reactivation is often less painful.

The characteristic lesions are small red papules, which develop into painful vesicles, sometimes confluent, after 36–72 hours (Figure 17.3 and Figure 17.4). These then dry up, crust over, and heal without leaving a scar. The pathognomonic morphology, differing from other genital ulcers, permits an easy diagnosis. Sometimes vulval oedema and inguinal lymph node enlargement occur. In reactivation, the clinical signs are more transient and difficult to diagnose so the history is very important.

Figure 17.3 Herpes simplex infection – multiple painful vesicles.

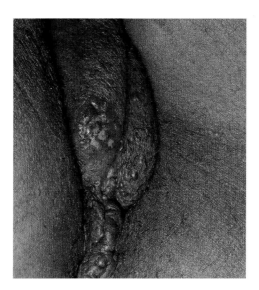

Figure 17.4 Confluent vesicles in HSV.

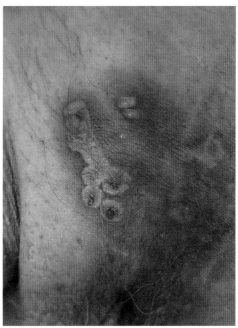

In patients who are immunosuppressed, HSV infection can have very atypical features. It is often hypertrophic (Figure 17.5) and may cause diagnostic difficulty as it can be mistaken for a tumour. These patients require prolonged courses of antiviral therapy to eradicate the lesions

Differential Diagnosis

The differential diagnosis of a vulval ulcer should always be taken into consideration; particularly aphthous ulcers, Behcet's disease, Crohn's disease, syphilis, chancroid, early neoplasia, excoriation and so forth (see Chapter 8). Varicella zoster and cytomegalovirus infection can look similar.

Diagnosis

The diagnosis may be made clinically but can be confirmed by viral swabs. These should be taken as soon as possible after the vesicles appear. Culture has a high sensitivity but PCR methods are better and are increasingly used. Serology may be helpful if swabs are negative but does not differentiate between types 1 and 2 of the virus.

Basic Management

The therapeutic approach depends on the type of infection (primary or reactivation). Oral treatment is preferred as topical treatment is not adequate. The administration of oral analgesics or topical local anaesthetic cream should be considered as the lesions are very painful.

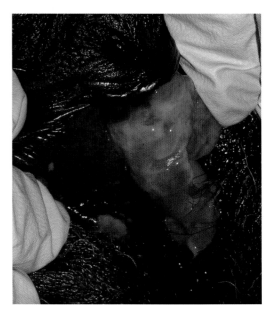

Figure 17.5 Hypertrophic HSV infection in immunosuppressed.

- **Primary infection**: aciclovir 400 mg three times a day; valaciclovir 500 mg twice a day, famciclovir 250 mg three times a day. Treatment should be continued until no new lesions appear which may be up to 10 days. Treatment of the primary infection does not seem to influence the pattern of reactivation or the number of recurrent episodes.
- **Reactivation**: recurrent episodes can have an impact on psychosexual health and general quality of life. Aciclovir 200 mg five times a day; valaciclovir 400 mg twice a day, or famciclovir 125 mg twice a day can be used for 5 days.If the patient is experiencing more than six episodes per year, suppressive therapy reducing the frequency of genital herpes recurrences by 70%–80% should be considered. Aciclovir 400 mg twice a day or valaciclovir 500 mg a day for 6 months are generally used.

HSV Infection and Pregnancy

Primary infection with HSV in pregnancy can cause important sequelae for the foetus including spontaneous miscarriage (25% cases), preterm delivery (75% cases < 37 weeks), low foetal weight, retinitis or mucous / skin infection (45%), encephalitis (33%), disseminated disease (22%) with neurological sequelae in more than 50% of neonates.

Eighty-five per cent of cases of transmission occur during delivery due to the prolonged contact with vaginal infected secretions. In the post partum period (8–10%) infection occurs for the same reason. The persistence of HSV in vaginal secretions (viral shedding) occurs easily due to the physiological reduction in immune-competence in pregnancy. Transmission before delivery can occur rarely in 5–8% of cases by vertical transplacental transfer or by contamination from the uterine cervix. There are no differences in HSV neonatal vertical transmission between women treated with aciclovir and the general population.

It has been shown that intra partum transmission occurs in 70% of cases without any symptoms or clinical lesions. It is recommended that those with a history of recurrent infection use aciclovir from 36 weeks gestation, to reduce the development of the lesions. Delivery by Caesarean section is recommended in the presence of clinical lesions and in those developing a primary infection in the last trimester of pregnancy as the risk of transmission is highest at this time.

Further Reading

Garland, S. M. and Steben, M. (2014) Genital herpes. *Best Practice and Research: Clinical Obstetrics and Gynaecology* **28**, 1098–1110.

Gupta, R., Warren, T. and Wald, A. (2007) Genital herpes. *Lancet* **370**, 2127–2137.

Patel, R., Green, J., Clarke, E. *et al.* (2014) UK national guideline of the management of anogenital herpes. *International Journal of STD and AIDS.* doi: 10.1177/0956462415580512

Stephenson-Farry, A. and Gardella, C. (2014) Herpes simplex infection during pregnancy. *Obstetrics and Gynecology Clinics of North America* **41**, 601–614.

Useful Web Sites for Patient Information

British Association for Sexual Health and HIV:
http://www.bashh.org/documents/HSV_2014%20IJSTDA.pdf (accessed 14 September 2016)
http://www.bashh.org/documents/HSV%20PIL%202015%20Screen-friendly.pdf (accessed 14 September 2016)

CDC guidelines on treatment of genital herpes:
http://www.cdc.gov/std/tg2015/herpes.htm (accessed 14 September 2016)

International Society for the Study of Vulvovaginal Disease
http://www.issvd.org/3471/ (accessed 18 September 2016)

Royal College of Obstetricians and Gynaecologists guidelines on management of herpes infection in pregnancy:
https://www.rcog.org.uk/globalassets/documents/guidelines/management-genital-herpes.pdf (accessed 14 September 2016)

Human Papillomavirus Infection

Human papillomavirus (HPV) is responsible for the development of a multitude of diseases affecting the lower genital tract in women. 40 different HPV types may affect the ano-genital area. The prevalence of HPV infection is highest in women aged 17–33 years with a peak of incidence in the 20-24 year age group. HPV infection can be asymptomatic, subclinical, or transient. They are small nonenveloped DNA viruses that infect the basal layers of the skin and mucosal surfaces.

Depending on the viral type, host immune response, and local environmental factors, HPV infection is responsible for condyloma acuminata (genital warts), undifferentiated vulval intraepithelial neoplasia (VIN), or certain types of squamous cell carcinoma (SCC). Condylomata are the result of low-risk HPV infection (90% are associated with HPV types 6 and 11) and have virtually no risk of neoplastic progression. Most infections will spontaneously clear within 12–18 months so the immune system has an important role. Patients who are immunosuppressed often have much more severe infections, which are more challenging to treat. They are also at higher risk of developing malignancy.

Epidemiology

HPV infection is one of the most common sexually transmitted disease with approximately 500 000–1 million new cases diagnosed each year in the United States. The incidence of condylomata has increased since 1980. HPV is a very contagious virus with reported transmission rates of 65%. The median time between infection and development of lesions is about 5–6 months among women. Risk factors for condylomata include:

- Infection with HPV types 6 and 11.
- A large number of sexual partners.
- Unprotected intercourse.
- A history of other sexually transmitted infections.
- Smoking.
- The use of oral contraceptives.
- Immunodeficiency. In particular, immunosuppression during pregnancy may cause reactivation of latent infection and the risk of developing condyloma acuminata in pregnancy is doubled.

Pathophysiology

It is important to distinguish the two biological sequences once HPV has entered into the basal layer of the squamous epithelium. The first biological behaviour is that of a "latent infection" in which HPV DNA persists in the basal cells without replication. In this case HPV can only by identified using molecular detection. The second biological behaviour is a 'productive infection'. The HPV DNA replication occurs in the intermediate and superficial layers of the squamous epithelium. The viral proliferation causes the typical morphological wart appearance, known as 'koilocytic change'.

The Concept of Vulval Subclinical Lesion

The concept of a subclinical lesion is based on the integration of cytological and histological studies previously and molecular biology technology more recently, together with colposcopic observation on the cervix. This led to a new interpretation of colposcopic, histological and cytological features, classified in the past as 'low grade dysplasia' and thereafter as subclinical infection or 'HPV cervical presence'. Translating the colposcopic concepts and acetic acid application from cervix and vagina to the vulva has shown how, on the vulva, the reaction of papilla-like structures to acetic acid was possible; this phenomenon was described as subclinical vulval lesions, HPV- related. However, for the correct clinical diagnosis and management, it is essential to understand vestibular papillomatosis as a normal anatomical variant on the vulva (see Chapter 1). Vestibular papillomatosis is the presence (usually in the vestibule only), of papillomata covered by squamous epithelium very similar to that covering the vestibule. These structures were described by Buschke in 1909 as the female equivalent of the pearly coronal papules seen on the penis. Other terms were therefore used to describe this condition. The presence of such papillomas was described first by Altemeyer in 1982 as 'hirsuties papillaris vulvae'. In 1983 Friedrich called them 'papilla vestibularis' and, until the 1990s, the theory that these were of viral origin prevailed. A large number of healthy women who just had this normal anatomical variant were treated for HPV infection by destructive methods to remove the lesions. The theory that they were due to a sexually transmitted infection led to psychological issues with feelings of guilt and fear about carrying an oncogenic virus. Vestibular papillomatosis is now known to be an anatomical variant, and not caused by HPV.

Histology

Condylomata show papillomatosis with inward bending of the rete ridges. Basal and parabasal hyperplasia are usually present with accentuation of the intercellular bridges of the keratinocytes. The koilocytic change is where keratinocytes have perinuclear clearing and enlarged nuclei that may be hyperchromatic. However, the finding of koilocytosis is not diagnostic of HPV infection and the loss of glycogen when the sections are processed can lead to vacuolated cells that resemble koilocytes. This is a particular issue in vestibular biopsies.

Clinical Features

Genital warts are usually asymptomatic. Some patients describe non-specific symptoms of pruritus, burning and soreness. The incubation period can be up to 18 months and some patients will have lesions that resolve spontaneously without them ever being aware of them.

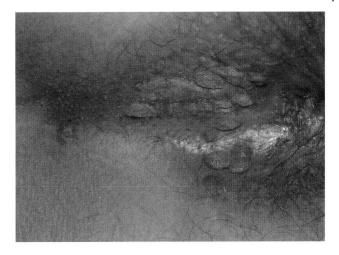

Figure 17.6 Warts – papillomatous lesions.

An HPV infection can manifest in several ways. The typical clinical lesion is the *condyloma acuminatum*, with a pedunculated appearance, an irregular and hyperkeratotic surface with variable dimensions and often multicentric (Figure 17.6).

Another lesion is the *condyloma planum,* a round plane lesion, sometimes raised but with a pleated surface. In general, this kind of condyloma is multiple and separated from healthy skin or mucosa. The papular lesions can merge together forming plaques (Figure 17.7).

The *condyloma papillomatosus* is a sessile lesion, which can be single or multiple, formed by papillae, merging together with a large base. When localized at a mucosal site they can have a vascular supply.

The commonest site is on the vulva but the vagina, cervix and perianal skin may also be affected. Lesions can also occur on the oral mucosa and pharynx.

Diagnosis

Diagnosis can be made via direct visual inspection. This may be helped by magnification and bright lighting, especially in the case of smaller lesions.

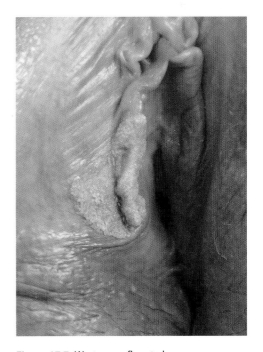

Figure 17.7 Warts – confluent plaques.

The use of the colposcope and acetic acid adds little to naked-eye examination of the vulva. If the diagnosis is uncertain or a VIN is suspected then a biopsy is needed. When a patient is diagnosed with genital warts she should undergo testing for other sexually transmitted infection as well as cervical cytology screening. Latent infection cannot be diagnosed except for molecular biology techniques detecting HPV-DNA.

Treatment

In the natural course of the disease, if left untreated, 30-40% of genital warts will spontaneously resolve. However, some will remain unchanged and others will increase in size and / or number.

The most common treatments are painful and nonspecific, removing the clinically evident lesions rather than eliminating the HPV viral infection.

Available therapeutic approaches involve pharmacological tissue destruction (podophyllotoxin, bichloroacetic acid / tri-chloroacetic acid), immune modulation (imiquimod, sinecatechins) or surgical excision procedures. Therapy options vary in terms of dosing, discomfort, pain, cost, duration of therapy and success rates. At this time, no evidence exists to recommend one therapy as superior over others. The choice of treatment is based on patient and / or provider preference, size / location of warts, cost of treatment, convenience, and experienced adverse effects. There is a high incidence of recurrence (13–65%) with condylomata, and multiple treatments and / or use of multiple therapeutic modalities is often required.

HPV Vaccine

There are two established vaccines (quadrivalent and bivalent) which have been evaluated in large trials and shown to dramatically reduce the incidence of genital warts. These are now given routinely in many countries as part of vaccination programmes and their increasing use should reduce the overall burden of disease from these viruses.

Genital Warts in Children

Although HPV can be transmitted by nonsexual routes, it is always important to consider the possibility of sexual abuse when genital warts are seen in children. A specialized paediatrician should always be involved in investigation and management.

Further Reading

Garland, S. M., Hernandez-Avila, M., Wheeler, S. M. *et al.* (2007) Quadrivalent vaccine against human papilloma virus to prevent ano-genital diseases. *New England Journal of Medicine* **356**, 1928–1943.

Steben, M. and Garland, S. M. (2014) Genital warts. *Best Practice and Research: Clinical Obstetrics and Gynecology* **28**, 1063–1073.

Useful Web Sites for Patient Information

CDC guidance:
http://www.cdc.gov/std/tg2015/warts.htm (accessed 14 September 2016)

UK national guideline on the management of anogenital warts 2015:
http://www.bashh.org/documents/UK%20national%20guideline%20on%20Warts%202015%20FINAL.pdf (accessed 14 September 2016)

Molluscum Contagiosum

Molluscum contagiosum is caused by a pox virus. These infections are not serious and disappear without treatment but can last for 12–18 months. They are spread from person to person by touching the affected skin and self-inoculation is possible.

Symptoms

The lesions are rarely painful but they may itch. Scratching can lead to spread of the molluscum infection, secondary bacterial infection or scarring.

Clinical Appearance

The lesions have very characteristic features. They are flesh-coloured, dome-shaped papules, pearly in appearance. They are usually 1–5 mm in diameter, with a typical dimpled or umbilicated centre (Figure 17.8). Occasionally a giant, solitary molluscum lesion can develop. In about 10% of the cases, eczema develops around the lesions. This is a particular feature as the lesion self-resolves and an inflammatory reaction develops as a result of host immunity.

Diagnosis

The diagnosis is made on the clinical appearance and diagnostic tests are unnecessary. The virus cannot routinely be cultured. Sometimes there can be clinical doubt with the giant solitary lesions and the diagnosis can then be confirmed by excisional biopsy.

Histologically, molluscum contagiosum is characterized by molluscum bodies in the epidermis above the basal layer. These are large cells with abundant granular eosinophilic cytoplasm (accumulated virions), and a small peripheral nucleus.

Treatment

No treatment is needed as the lesions will eventually resolve spontaneously. However, they can be treated with cryotherapy or laser therapy. Cantharidin – a chemical compound secreted by some species of beetles – and imiquimod are alternatives but these can cause irritant side effects on the vulva.

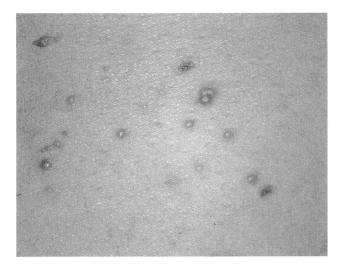

Figure 17.8 Molluscum contagiosum – umbilicated papules.

Further Reading

Fernando, I., Pritchard, J., Edwards, S. K. and Grover, D. (2014) UK national guideline for the management of molluscum in adults 2014. *International Journal of STD and AIDS*. doi:10.1177/0956462414554435

Useful Web Site for Patient Information

British Association for Sexual Health and HIV:
http://www.bashh.org/documents/MC_2014%20IJSTDA.pdf (accessed 14 September 2016)

Scabies

Scabies is caused by the *Sarcoptes scabei* mite and is transmitted by close contact, including sexual contact. It is not common on the vulva. Crusted or Norwegian scabies is a severe infection with thousands of mites present on the skin and is usually seen in the immunosuppressed. It is highly infectious.

Clinical Features

The characteristic clinical sign is the burrow, which is usually seen on the hands or soles (Figure 17.9). There is frequently an associated eczematous response and the excoriation may make the burrows difficult to see on the vulva.

Diagnosis

The diagnosis is clinical but can be confirmed by extracting a mite from a burrow. The mites may also be visible with the dermatoscope, but this is not a practical technique on the vulva.

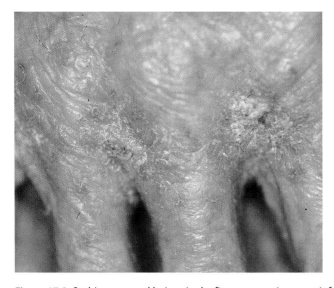

Figure 17.9 Scabies – crusted lesions in the finger spaces in severe infection.

Treatment

Permethrin 5% cream or malathion 0.5% solution should be applied from the neck down and left on for 12 hours. A second application should be used 7 days later. Systemic ivermectin 200micrograms/kg is very effective and can be used in crusted scabies.

Further Reading

Rosamilia, L. (2014) Scabies. *Seminars in Cutaneous Medicine and Surgery* **33**, 106–109.
Currie, B. J. and McCarthy, J. S. (2010) Permethrin and ivermectin for scabies. *New England Journal of Medicine* **362**, 717–725.

Useful Web Site for Patient Information

British Association of Dermatologists:
http://www.bad.org.uk/shared/get-file.ashx?id=127&itemtype=document (accessed 14 September 2016)

Pubic lice

Infection with the crab louse *Phthirus pubis* infests the pubic hair and frequently occurs with other STIs.

Clinical Features

There is severe itching and there may be a secondary eczematous reaction. The lice can also attach to the eyelashes.

Treatment

Permethrin 5% or malathion are used as treatment. Eyelashes can be treated with a paraffin based ointment.

Useful Web Site for Patient Information

UK National Guidelines on Phthirus Pubis Infection 2007:
http://www.bashh.org/documents/28/28.pdf (accessed 14 September 2016)

18

Vulval Infection – Nonsexually Transmitted

The two most common vulval infections not transmitted via a sexual route are candidiasis and bacterial vaginosis. In both cases, the normal balance of the flora of the vulva and vagina is upset, causing overgrowth of organisms leading to symptoms.

However, there are several less common infections that occur on the vulva that are not transmitted via sexual contact. Many of these are rare in the developed world but are listed in Table 18.1. Advice should be sought from experts in tropical medicine regarding diagnosis and management where relevant.

Bacterial Infections

- Bacterial vaginosis.
- Erythrasma.
- Staphylococcal and streptococcal infection.

Bacterial Vaginosis

Bacterial vaginosis (BV) is the commonest cause of a vaginal discharge in women during the reproductive years and is due to an imbalance in the normal flora causing overgrowth of *Gardnerella vaginalis.* It has been associated with pre-term birth and endometritis.

Clinical Features

The classic feature is of an offensive profuse vaginal discharge. Inflammation is not generally associated, but the discharge can cause an irritant vulval dermatitis in some women.

Diagnosis

The Amsel diagnostic criteria include a white discharge, vaginal pH .4.5, clue cells on direct microscopy and a fishy odour with the addition of 10% potassium hydroxide.

Treatment

Metronidazole or clindamycin are recommended.

A Practical Guide to Vulval Disease: Diagnosis and Management, First Edition. Fiona Lewis, Fabrizio Bogliatto and Marc van Beurden.
© 2017 John Wiley & Sons Ltd. Published 2017 by John Wiley & Sons Ltd.

Table 18.1 Nonsexually transmitted vulval infections.

		Clinical features	Diagnosis	Treatment
Nematode infection	Threadworm infection (*Enterobius vermicularis*)	Common infection in children; anal and vulval pruritus	Identification of the threadworms or eggs on perianal skin – can be seen by applying adhesive tape to the skin and examining microscopically	Piperazine or mebendazole
	Filariasis[a]	Lymphoedema and elephantiasis	Histology	Diethylcarbazine in increasing doses. Surgery may be required
Trematode (fluke) infection	Schistosomiasis[a]	Usually occurs before puberty with granulomatous nodules; swelling and scarring can occur	Ova are seen in the urine. ELISA tests available	Praziquantel
Protozoa	Leishmaniasis[a]	Large ulcers that can be similar to those seen in syphilis or donovanosis	Histology or specialized culture	Sodium stilbogluconate or antimony preparations
	Amoebiasis[a] caused by *Entamoeba histolytica*	Abscesses on vulva, perineum or cervix with lymphadenopathy	Amoebae may be seen in the ulcers or on scrapings from cervix	Metronidazole
Mycobacterial infection	Tuberculosis[a]	Vulval involvement less common than upper genital tract; nodules, ulcers and scars occur; more common in immunosuppressed patients	Histology	Antituberculous treatment
	Leprosy[a]	Can be direct inoculation of the vulva or involvement by haematogenous spread		Expert advice
Other bacterial infections	Actinomycosis	Actinomycosis species can infect intrauterine devices	Culture and histology	Penicillin is first line, but Tetracyclines, clindamycin and erythromycin are alternative treatments.
	Mycoplasma	Ureaplasma and mycoplasma species may be found in the vagina in asymptomatic patients; Bartholin's abscesses may occur	Culture and histology	As for actinomycosis

Note:
[a]Ask for expert advice on investigation and management.

Further Reading

Donders, G., Zodzika, J. and Rezeberga, D. (2014) Treatment of bacterial vaginosis: what we have and what we miss. *Expert Opinion on Pharmacotherapy* **15**, 645–657.

Useful Web Sites for Patient Information

BASHH patient information:
http://www.bashh.org/documents/BV%20PIL%20Screen%20-%20Edit.pdf (accessed 14 September 2016)

CDC guidance:
http://www.cdc.gov/std/tg2015/bv.htm (accessed 14 September 2016)

UK National Guideline for the Management of Bacterial Vaginosis 2012:
http://www.bashh.org/documents/4413.pdf (accessed 14 September 2016)

Erythrasma

Erythrasma is an infection caused by *Corynebacterium minutissimum,* a Gram-positive aerobic bacterium It is found on normal skin but particularly favours moist environments, therefore vulval involvement is common. Predisposing factors include immunosuppression, diabetes and obesity.

Clinical Features

The areas are well demarcated (Figure 18.1) with superficial scaling at the edge (Figure 18.2). There may be a red / brown discoloration to the plaques with lesions at other sites, including the axillae and under the breasts.

Differential Diagnosis

Tinea cruris is the major differential diagnosis and the two infections can sometimes occur together.

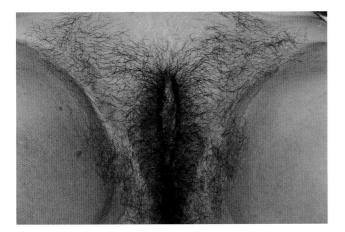

Figure 18.1 Erythrasma.

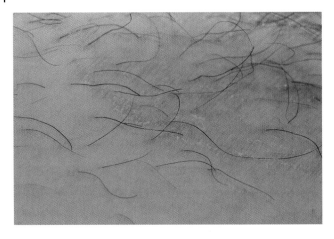

Figure 18.2 Scaly edge to the plaques.

Table 18.2 Staphylococcal and streptococcal infections.

Staphylococcus	Streptococcus	Either
Folliculitis	Streptococcal perianal dermatitis	Cellulitis
Bartholin's gland abscess	Necrotizing fasciitis	
Toxic shock syndrome		
Staphylococcal scalded skin syndrome		

Diagnosis

Microscopy of skin scrapings (see Chapter 5) can identify the organism. The diagnosis can also be made by using a Wood's lamp as affected areas will show a coral-pink fluorescence due to the presence of a porphyrin.

Basic Management

Topical treatment with fusidic acid cream or topical erythromycin may be effective. Oral erythromycin 250 mg four times a day for 2 weeks is used in more severe infections.

Useful Web Site for Patient Information

DermNet:
http://www.dermnetnz.org/bacterial/erythrasma.html (accessed 14 September 2016)

Staphylococcal and Streptococcal Infections

These two common pathogenic bacteria cause a range of clinical patterns of infection (see Table 18.2).

Folliculitis

Staphyloccous aureus is the usual agent responsible for folliculitis, a pustular infection around hair follicles, boils and abscesses. The increasingly recognized variant of *S. aureus*, PVL (Panton Leucocidin Valentine) can cause infection in the vulval area.

Pathophysiology

A short-lived pseudofolliculitis is common after shaving or waxing to remove the pubic hair. This is an inflammatory response to the trauma of hair removal. However, infective folliculitis is persistent, especially in diabetics and those who are immunosuppressed. Acute lesions are superficial but deeper infections may cause intrafollicular abscesses and fibrotic inflammation.

Clinical Features

Small pustular lesions with surrounding inflammation are seen. These are centred on hair follicles (Figure 18.3).

Diagnosis

Microscopy and culture of swabs taken from active lesions will demonstrate the organisms. If the patient has recurrent infections it is helpful to check swabs from other body sites such as the nose, axillae and groin as they may be staphylococcal carriers.

Basic Management

Topical antiseptics used as a wash, for example 1% chlorhexidine gluconate, and a short course of a topical antibiotic can be used in minor infections. Oral treatment may be needed and a tetracycline (e.g. lymecycline, 408 mg, once daily) or erythromycin 500 mg twice daily for 3 months, may be required.

Further Reading

Fogo, A., Kemp, N. and Morris-Jones, R. (2011) PVL positive Staphylococcus aureus skin infections. *British Medical Journal* **9**, 343.

Bartholin Abscess

A Bartholin abscess occurs when the duct from the gland becomes blocked. Fluid in the gland builds up and may become infected. This fluid may accumulate over many years before an abscess occurs. They may recur. Common organisms causing infection are *s. aureus* and *Streptococcus faecalis*.

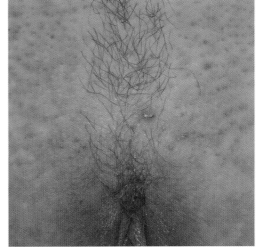

Figure 18.3 Folliculitis.

Clinical Features

Often the abscess appears quickly over several days. The area will become very hot and swollen. Walking, sitting and any activity that puts pressure on the vulva, such as intercourse, will cause severe pain. A tender lump on either side of the vaginal opening, usually seen on the lower third, is visible (Figure 18.4). There may be associated fever and malaise.

Differential Diagnosis

Other benign lesions such as hidradenoma papilliferum, lipomas, epidermoid cysts can look similar but these should be asymptomatic.

Basic Management

The first step is soaking in warm water four times a day for several days. This can ease the discomfort and can help the abscess open and drain on its own. Surgical management, together with appropriate antibiotics, may be required.

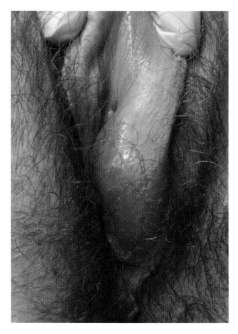

Figure 18.4 Bartholin's abscess.

Drainage of the Abscess

Incision and drainage through a small surgical opening will relieve symptoms. The procedure can be done under local anaesthesia in an outpatient setting. Simple aspiration of the cyst can be helpful as this reduces the size and relieves symptoms quickly. A Penrose drainage tube may be inserted and left in place to allow draining while the area heals. Soaking in warm water can then begin 1–2 days afterwards. Sexual intercourse should be avoided until the catheter is removed.

Marsupialization

Women can also be treated with this minimal surgical procedure when there are more than two or three recurrences of the abscess. The procedure involves creating a small, permanent opening to help the gland drain. It can sometimes be done in an outpatient setting but in other cases it will need to be done in hospital under general anaesthesia. This treatment has demonstrated a healing time of less than 2 weeks. No recurrence was observed in any studies with marsupialization. However, when compared with patients treated by incision and drainage before primary closure, patients with marsupialization healed significantly more slowly (1 to 21 days versus 3 to 11 days). There were no significant differences in abscess recurrence.

After marsupialisation, it is recommended soaking the area in warm water 1–2 days afterward. Oral analgesia should be prescribed. Sexual intercourse should be avoided for 4 weeks after surgery.

The prognosis is excellent, but the abscess may recur in about 1 in 10 cases. It is important to treat any vaginal infection that is diagnosed at the same time as the abscess.

Further Reading

Wechter, M.E., Wu, J. M., Marzano, D. and Haefner, H. (2009) Management of Bartholin duct cysts and abscesses: a systematic review. *Obstetrical and Gynecological Survey* **64**, 395–404.

Yuk, J. S., Kim, Y. J., Hur, J. Y. and Shin, J. H. (2013) Incidence of Bartholin duct cysts and abscesses in the Republic of Korea. *International Journal of Gynecology and Obstetrics* **122**, 62–64.

Other Staphylococcal Infections

Toxic Shock Syndrome

Menstrual toxic shock syndrome is caused by toxins released from *S. aureus*. It was associated with retained tampons but is now rare.

Staphylococcal Scalded Skin Syndrome

This is an infection mediated by toxins produced by *S. aureus*. It is more common in children and superficial desquamation occurs (Figure 18.5). The flexural areas may be the first to be involved before spread to other areas. Flucloaxacillin is the treatment of choice.

Cellulitis

Group B streptococcal species are frequent commensals in the vagina. However, those of Group A are responsible for more serious infections such as cellulitis.

Clinical Features

There is rapid spread of painful erythema, which can affect all areas of the vulva and spread to the groins and perianal area (Figure 18.6). Oedema, with or without blistering, is common. The patient is unwell with fever and systemic symptoms. It most commonly follows trauma or surgery.

Diagnosis

The diagnosis is clinical but swabs taken from the area, especially from any broken areas of skin, may demonstrate the causative organism. Blood cultures may be positive in severe infections.

Differential Diagnosis

Pyoderma gangrenosum is an inflammatory condition where deep ulceration occurs rapidly. There is a purple edge to the ulcers.

Other Streptococcal Infections

Streptococcal dermatitis usually affects the anogenital area of children and is much more common in males.

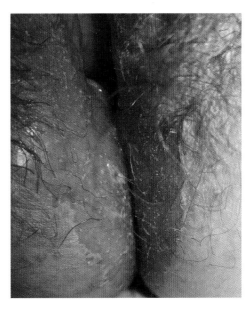

Figure 18.5 Staphylococcal infection (*S. aureus*) with superficial desquamation.

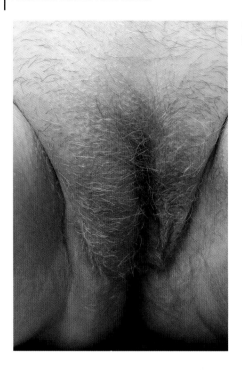

Figure 18.6 Vulval cellulitis with erythema and oedema involving the right labium majus and extending to mons pubis.

Necrotising fasciitis (synergistic bacterial gangrene). This severe, rapidly extending and life-threatening disease is caused by multiple bacteria, which act synergistically causing widespread infection. Anaerobes may also be involved. Immediate surgical debridement is vital.

Further Reading

Holtzman, L. C., Hitti, E. and Harrow, J. (2013) Incision and drainage, in *Clinical Procedures in Emergency Medicine*, 5th edn (eds J. R. Roberts and J. R. Hedges). Elsevier, Philadelphia, PA.

Wood, S. C. (2015) Clinical manifestations and therapeutic management of vulvar cellulitis and abscess: methicillin resistant staphylococcal aureus, necrotising fasciitis, Bartholin abscess, Crohn disease of the vulva, hidradenitis suppurativa. *Clinical Obstetrics and Gynecology* **58**, 503–511.

Vulvovaginal Candidiasis

Candida species are part of the normal flora of the vulva and vagina and they are rarely found on the vulva in isolation. Vulval infection therefore usually occurs after a vaginal or perineal infection.

Pathophysiology

Candida albicans is responsible for 90% of cases but other species include *C. glabrata, C. tropicalis* and *C. krusei.* These may be more resistant to treatment.

It is important to ask about any risk factors that can be corrected. These include diabetes, obesity, pregnancy, systemic antibiotic or steroid medication, immunosuppression and hygiene habits. The older high oestrogen containing oral contraceptives were also associated with candidiasis but with the use of the newer low-dosage oral contraceptives this is no longer thought to be a major risk factor.

Clinical Features

Itching, with resultant excoriation due to rubbing and scratching, is the most frequent symptom. Symptoms are worse with micturition, sexual intercourse and the use of tight-fitting clothes. Some women develop similar symptoms with pruritus before menstruation and this is associated with dyspareunia. Swabs are not always positive and topical treatment resolves 90% of cases.

On examination, the clinical signs are variable depending on the entity and duration of infection.

The acute form is characterized by mucocutaneous erythema (Figure 18.7), oedema and a white, 'cottage-cheese'-like discharge. The lesions often involve the genito-crural folds, which develop superficial fissures. In widespread infection, the inner thighs develop erythema and small pustules (satellite lesions) (Figure 18.8).

In the chronic form, erythema is less evident but mild oedema of the labia minora and clitoris persists together with hypertrophy of the free edges of the labia majora and the perianal area as a result of continuous scratching. The typical discharge is absent.

Recurrent vulvovaginal candidiasis is defined as four or more episodes occurring in one year and the causative organism may be a nonalbicans type. The reasons for recurrent infection is not known but host immunity is probably important.

Differential Diagnosis

The differential diagnosis for candidiasis is wide and includes contact dermatitis (irritant or allergic), psoriasis, lichen planus, erysipelas, seborrhoeic dermatitis and Paget's disease. Many patients are assumed to have recurrent candidiasis without proper evaluation and many important dermatoses can be missed when a full assessment is not made.

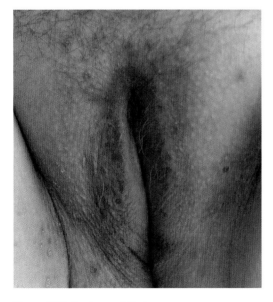

Figure 18.7 Acute candidiasis.

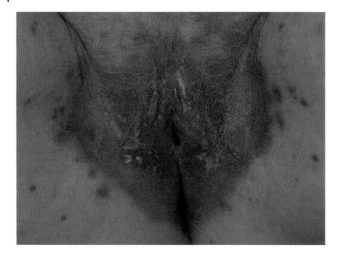

Figure 18.8 Satellite lesions spreading to thighs.

Diagnosis

In simple cases, the diagnosis may be clinical but, in patients with recurrent symptoms, it must be confirmed. Microscopy of a vaginal smear will demonstrate the hyphae. The pH of vaginal secretions is normal in candidiasis.

Treatment

Treatment should be aimed at the vulva and vagina. There is no need to treat the sexual partner. Topical treatment is based on imidazole formulations in noncomplicated infection. Vaginal therapy (cream or pessaries) can be used for 3–14 days but single-dose administration is also possible and many regimens are published in guidelines. The vulval treatment also lasts 3–14 days, using azole compounds. Other preparations include ciclopiroxolamine, nystatin and boric acid. Boric acid pessaries seem to be useful especially in imidazole resistant forms but are not readily available in Europe.

Oral treatment for both vaginal and vulval infection is preferable especially in those who have secondary inflammatory change as it avoids irritation from further topical treatment. Itraconazole 200 mg once a day for 4 days, or fluconazole, 150 mg in one dose, are used.

In those with recurrent candidiasis, long-term treatment with weekly doses of fluconazole, 150 mg, is helpful. This may be required for 3–6 months.

In pregnancy the use of topical azoles is recommended as they have no teratogenic risk.

Further Reading

Sobel, J. (2015) Recurrent vulvovaginal candidiasis. *American Journal of Obstetrics and Gynecology.* doi: 10.1016/j.ajog.2015.06.067

Useful Web Sites for Patient Information

CDC guidance:
http://www.cdc.gov/std/tg2015/candidiasis.htm (accessed 14 September 2016)

International Society for Study of Vulvovaginal Disease:
http://www.issvd.org/candidiasisyeast-infection/ (accessed 18 September 2016)

UK National Guidelines 2007:
http://www.bashh.org/documents/1798.pdf (accessed 14 September 2016)

Tinea Cruris

Tinea cruris is a dermatophyte fungal infection that can affect the inguinal folds, buttocks and vulva. It is less common in women than men.

Pathophysiology

The common species are *Trichophyton rubrum and Epidermophyton flocculosum.* The environmental factors of moisture, warmth and occlusion in the genital area predispose to the infection.

Clinical Features

The classic features are a well defined scaly eruption, which gradually spreads out with central sparing (Figure 18.9). It may be itchy but may not cause any symptoms at all.

It is very important to consider the diagnosis when folliculitic lesions are seen as the typical appearances are often lost if the patient has used a topical steroid, when it has been mistaken for an eczematous eruption. This is known as 'tinea incognito' (Figure 18.10) and presents with inflammatory papular lesions (see Chapter 6).

Differential Diagnosis

Candidiasis, eczema, erythrasma and flexural psoriasis can look similar.

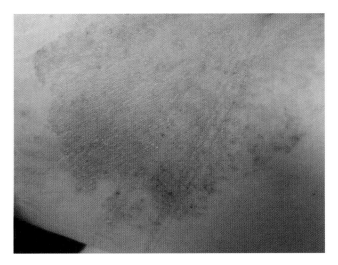

Figure 18.9 Tinea cruris – extending lesions with central sparing.

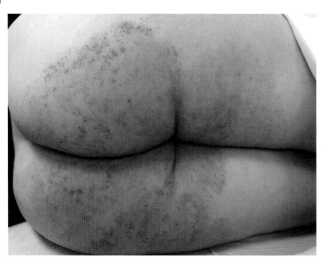

Figure 18.10 Extensive infection caused by inappropriate use of topical steroids (tinea incognito).

Diagnosis

Skin scrapings (see Chapter 5) are taken for microscopy and culture.

Basic Management

In a non-hair-bearing area, a topical antifungal preparation is adequate. It can be applied twice daily for a few weeks until the eruption resolves. In a hair-bearing area such as the outer labia majora, a systemic agent is likely to be needed. Oral terbinafine, 250 mg/day, or itraconazole, 200 mg, twice daily for 2–4 weeks, are effective.

Further Reading

Eckert, L. O. and Lentz, G. M. (2013) Infections of the lower genital tract: vulva, vagina, cervix, toxic shock syndrome, endometritis, and salpingitis, in *Comprehensive Gynecology*, 6th edn (eds G. M. Lentz, R. A. Lobo, D. M. Gershenson and V. L. Katz). Elsevier, Philadelphia, PA.

El-Gohary, M., van Zuuren, E. J., Fedorowicz, Z. *et al.* (2014) Topical antifungal treatments for tines cruris and tinea corporis. *Cochrane Database of Systematic Reviews* **8** (Art. No.L CD009992).

Useful Web Site for Patient Information

DermNet:
http://dermnetnz.org/fungal/tinea-cruris.html (accessed 14 September 2016)

Viral Infections

Varicella Zoster (Shingles)

This occurs when the varicella virus is reactivated after previous chickenpox infections. It is most common in the elderly and immunosuppressed and if lesions are seen on the vulva if the S3 dermatome is involved. There may be a painful prodrome before vesicles appear, which then crust over. Lymphadenopathy is frequent. Urinary retention and postherpetic neuralgia are complications.

19

Vulval Intraepithelial Neoplasia

Introduction

Vulval intraepithelial neoplasia (VIN) is a squamous precancerous condition. The nonsquamous types of VIN are extramammary Paget's disease (see Chapter 20) and melanoma *in situ* (see below). Squamous VIN can be divided into undifferentiated or usual VIN (uVIN) and differentiated VIN (dVIN). Undifferentiated VIN can be further classified into different subtypes – *warty* and *basaloid* (Table 19.1). The classification and terminology is evolving and a recent change has been accepted by the International Society for the Study of Vulvovaginal Disease (ISSVD). The purpose of this latest classification is to differentiate between the various types of intraepithelial lesions of the vulva, according to their etiologies (i.e. HPV or non-HPV related). Low-grade squamous intraepithelial lesions (LSIL) are not premalignant and therefore do not need to be treated to prevent progression. The previously used term 'VIN' is now reserved for premalignant lesions, which should be treated to prevent progression to cancer. Premalignant HPV related lesions are termed 'high-grade squamous intraepithelial lesions' (HSIL) and non-HPV related lesions are termed 'differentiated type'.

Epidemiology

Undifferentiated VIN mainly affects young women, is caused by human papilloma virus (HPV) infection and therefore usually presents as a multifocal disease on the vulva and is often associated with other intraepithelial neoplasia in the lower genital tract. Recurrences after treatment occur in up to 50% of women and are associated with smoking, immunosuppression, multifocality, positive surgical margins and large lesion size. Since the 1970s, the incidence of uVIN has been estimated as 5 per 100 000 but it is increasing, particularly in the younger age group. This is most likely to be due to a rise in the incidence of HPV infection. Any age group is affected, but it is most common in women under 50. Most patients with uVIN are heavy smokers. Immunosuppression, such as HIV infection, or the use of immunosuppressant drugs, increases the risk of developing uVIN. Spontaneous regression of uVIN seldom occurs but when it does it is usually in women under 35 years, with multifocal pigmented lesions, and is often related to pregnancy.

Differentiated VIN is less common, although pathologists do recognize dVIN more often in recent years. Less than 2–5% of all VIN lesions are of the dVIN type. They are not related to HPV and are usually found in older women, observed in association with lichen sclerosus (LS). Differentiated VIN does not regress spontaneously.

A Practical Guide to Vulval Disease: Diagnosis and Management, First Edition. Fiona Lewis, Fabrizio Bogliatto and Marc van Beurden.
© 2017 John Wiley & Sons Ltd. Published 2017 by John Wiley & Sons Ltd.

Table 19.1 Squamous vulval intraepithelial neoplasia (VIN) terminology.

ISSVD, 1986	ISSVD, 2005	ISSVD, 2015
		Low-grade SIL (flat condyloma and HPV effect)
VIN 1, mild atypia	VIN, usual type (warty, basaloid, mixed)	High-grade SIL
VIN 2, moderate dysplasi		
VIN 3, severe dysplasia, CIS		
VIN 3, differentiated type	VIN, differentiated type	VIN, differentiated type

Aetiology

The lifetime risk of becoming infected with HPV in Western societies is around 80% and approximately 40% of all sexually active, female adolescents are infected with high-risk HPV (hrHPV) at least once. In less than 10% of cases, hrHPV persists and premalignant disorders of the lower anogenital tract, such as uVIN, can develop. The reported prevalence of HPV in VIN ranges from 72–100% and, in most cases, HPV16 is detected. HPV-DNA is found more commonly in multifocal VIN than in unifocal VIN and in VIN coexisting with other multicentric intraepithelial lesions in the lower genital tract.

In contrast to uVIN, the presence of HPV in dVIN is very rare and the exact cause of dVIN is still unclear. Differentiated VIN is related to LS and there is a clear relationship between dVIN and LS in skin adjacent to a vulval squamous cell carcinoma (SCC). Differentiated VIN is often HPV-negative and p53 positive.

Prevention

Undifferentiated VIN can be prevented by the use of the prophylactic quadrivalent HPV vaccine in girls, which provides sustained protection against uVIN. In the HPV-naïve population the vaccine efficacy against HPV16-18 related uVIN is nearly 95%. It is anticipated that a reduction in the precursor lesions of vulval cancer would reduce the rates of invasive vulval SCC.

It is assumed that prevention of dVIN and vulval SCC in patients with LS is best achieved by the use of ultrapotent corticosteroids.

Histological Features

Histopathologically, uVIN can be classified into different subtypes – *warty* and *basaloid* Both can be easily recognized. Typically, the epidermis is thickened and is accompanied by a surface reaction of hyperkeratosis and / or parakeratosis. There is loss of cell maturation with associated nuclear hyperchromasia, pleomorphism and numerous mitotic figures at all levels of the epidermis. The intraepithelial process may also involve the underlying skin appendages. The epidermis of *warty* VIN has wide and deep rete ridges, often reaching close to the surface, which gives a characteristic condylomatous appearance. There is striking cellular polymorphism and evidence for abnormal cell maturation. Koilocytosis, corps rounds, multinucleation, (abnormal) mitotic figures and acanthosis are common. *Basaloid* uVIN is characterized by a thickened epithelium with a relatively flat and nonpapillomatous surface. Large numbers of relative uniform undifferentiated cells with a basaloid appearance are seen in the epidermis. Mitotic figures are numerous but koilocytic cells and corps rounds are less frequently seen than in warty uVIN. Patterns of warty and basaloid uVIN are often found in the same lesion, which is referred to as *mixed* uVIN (Figure 19.1).

The histopathological diagnosis of dVIN is difficult and can be mistaken easily for a benign dermatosis because of the high degree of cellular differentiation and absence of widespread architectural disarray. Histopathological features are atypical mitoses in the basal layer, basal cellular atypia, dyskeratosis, prominent nucleoli and elongation and anastomosis of the rete ridges (Figure 19.2). Staining with MIB1 and p53 can be helpful in distinguishing dVIN from normal vulvar epithelium.

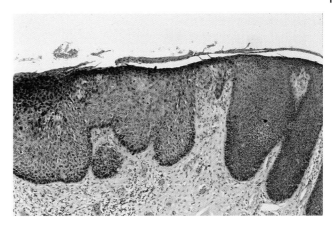

Figure 19.1 Undifferentiated VIN with, on the left, the warty type with the condylomatous appearance and the basaloid type with large numbers of relative uniform undifferentiated cells, on the right, often coexisting in one lesion.

Symptoms

Undifferentiated VIN causes many severe and long-lasting symptoms such as pruritus, vulvodynia and psychosexual dysfunction. Many patients experience episodes of anxiety and depression. However, a large proportion of women are without any vulval symptoms. As patients can be asymptomatic, accurate inspection of the vulva during routine gynaecological examination is important.

Clinical Features

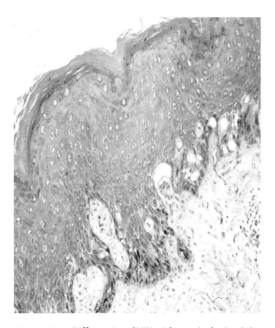

Figure 19.2 Differentiated VIN with atypical mitosis in the basal layer, basal cellular atypia, dyskeratosis, prominent nucleoli and elongation and anastomosis of the rete ridges.

Undifferentiated VIN has a variety of clinical appearances. Lesions are often multifocal, raised, well demarcated and asymmetrical. Lesions might be white, red or pigmented (Figure 19.3). The commonest affected sites are the labia majora and minora and the fourchette, but all sites of the vulva might be affected (Figure 19.4). Lesions may be subtle (Figure 19.5) or they can form large confluent plaques (Figure 19.6). Sometimes only

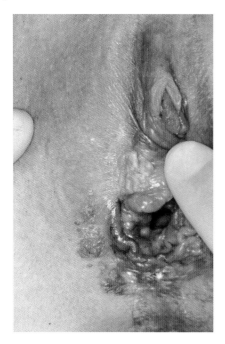

Figure 19.3 Typical multifocal uVIN with white, red and pigmented lesions.

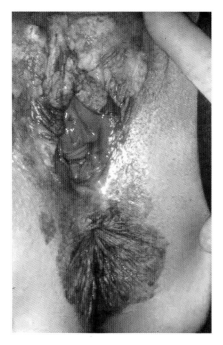

Figure 19.4 Extensive multifocal uVIN with perianal involvement.

Figure 19.5 Undifferentiated VIN with localized and small lesions.

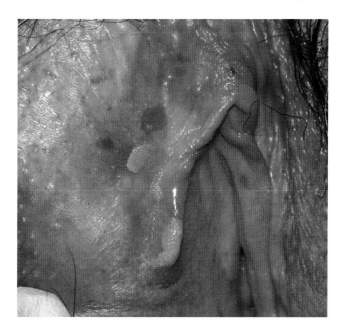

Figure 19.6 Multifocal uVIN lesions forming confluent plaques.

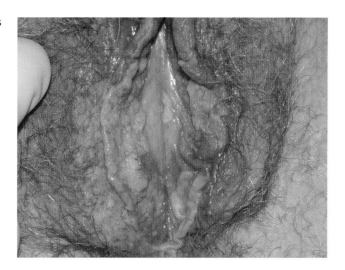

pigmented papules can be seen in young women – they can regress spontaneously (Figure 19.7). To confirm the diagnosis, a biopsy of the most suspicious part of the lesion should be performed under local anaesthesia. Over 80% of uVIN-affected women present with multifocal vulval disease, and often neoplastic changes can be found in the entire lower genital tract, namely anal intraepithelial neoplasia (AIN), perianal intraepithelial neoplasia (PAIN), vaginal intraepithelial neoplasia (VAIN) and cervical intraepithelial neoplasia (CIN).

Clinically, it is important to distinguish unifocal lesions from multifocal lesions, as unifocal VIN tends to progress to invasive carcinoma ten times more often than multifocal VIN does.

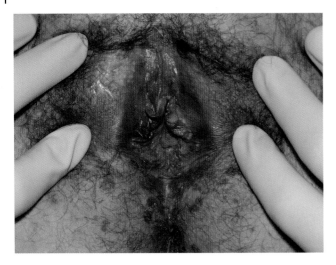

Figure 19.7 Undifferentiated VIN with only pigmented papules, also in the perianal region.

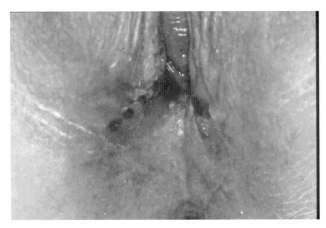

Figure 19.8 Differentiated VIN presenting with multifocal erosive lesions in the fourchette on the background of LS.

In addition, multicentric disease (lesions of cervix, vagina or anus) is common in uVIN patients and is age related, as it decreases from 60% in women under 35 years to 10% in women over 50 years of age. Therefore, a careful examination of the lower anogenital tract (vulva, perineum and perianal areas), which also includes the cervix and vagina, is mandatory.

Attention should be paid to the psychosexual consequences of uVIN and vulval excision. In general, surgical treatment of vulval lesions may lead to disfigurement, postoperative loss of quality of life and impaired sexual function. In addition, sexual function is correlated to the extent of excision. Therefore, treatments that preserve the anatomy of the vulva, such as imiquimod or CO_2-laser vaporization, can be important to prevent psychosexual sequelae.

Differentiated VIN is seldom diagnosed and then mostly as a solitary lesion. Patients are often symptomatic with a long-lasting history of LS or lichen planus (LP)-related symptoms of vulval itching and/or burning. It is commonly seen adjacent to LS and vulval SCC.

It can present as a grey-white hyperkeratotic area or as an erythematous or ulcerative lesion (Figure 19.8). Lesions are often unifocal and small. Because of the highly malignant potential of dVIN, any suspicious area in patients affected by LS or LP should be biopsied or excised without delay to obtain a representative histopathological diagnosis.

Management

There is a lack of consensus on the optimal surgical treatment method. The ideal management of women with VIN is complicated by the different age groups of women affected and the extent and occasional multifocal nature of this condition, which has a risk of recurrence of over 50%. The rationale nowadays for the treatment of uVIN is to treat the symptoms and exclude any underlying malignancy, with the continued aim of preserving the vulval anatomy and function. After having ruled out a vulval SCC by taking a biopsy or multiple biopsies there are different treatment options: cold-knife excision, CO_2 laser evaporization, cavitron ultrasonic surgical aspirator (CUSA), immune modulating drugs, imiquimod, antiviral drugs, such as cidofovir, experimental therapeutic HPV vaccines, photodynamic therapy or observation only.

For a long time, the choice of therapy for uVIN has been dominated by the premalignant nature of the disease. In the past, extensive surgery such as vulvectomy has been performed to remove the disease. Surgical treatment is effective in removing premalignant lesions but recurrence rates are high because persistent HPV infection is not affected by surgical treatment and surgical margins are often positive. In addition, one has to be aware that surgery can diminish the quality of life and sexual function because this is often associated with deformity and loss of vulval function, which has significant somatic and psychosexual morbidity, factors that need more consideration as uVIN is now being diagnosed in younger women. In 1995, Kaufman therefore addressed the importance of individualization of treatment, which should be directed towards preservation of the normal anatomy and function of the vulva. More limited surgery has been the approach in recent decades. Surgical treatment can be performed with different techniques. Cold-knife surgery or CO_2-laser evaporization have been used as a single technique or in combination. Laser evaporization can be an effective method in non-hair-bearing areas but because this technique destroys all tissue it is recommended that representative biopsies are taken beforehand. In surgery for uVIN there is only one trial comparing CO_2 laser surgery versus ultrasonic surgical aspirator (USA). These were equal in disease recurrence and side effects after one year. It has been demonstrated that taking multiple biopsies is a safe method to exclude invasive disease, and restricted surgery thereafter to be effective in relieving symptoms in multifocal VIN.

Although surgical excision remains the preferred method of care for small lesions, this is not suitable for the often multifocal and widespread uVIN, with its high recurrence rate and the mutilating effect of extensive surgery with the impaired effect on sexuality and quality of life. Less invasive medical interventions are indicated more for these lesions. The immunological aspects of uVIN, have increased the search for new immunotherapeutic approaches. The main advantages of medical treatment are preservation of vulval anatomy and function. Topical treatment is attractive because it can be applied directly by the patient and is easily monitored for efficacy. However, medical treatment does not provide a specimen for histological evaluation with the risk that early invasion is overlooked. For that reason, taking accurate biopsies is important before starting medical treatment. The use of 5-fluorouracil, bleomycin and trinitrochlorobenzene, which have been applied topically in the past, has been abandoned due to inefficacy and unacceptable side effects. Interferon-α therapy (IFN-α), which had promising results initially, is now limited in use due to side effects and high cost.

Imiquimod, a topical immune response modifier, which acts by binding on toll-like receptors (TLRs) on the cell surface of dendritic cells, thereby inducing secretion of pro-inflammatory cytokines, is approved for the treatment of genital wart. Undifferentiated VIN is an unlicensed indication for the use of imiquimod. However, in a systematic review, complete regression was observed in 26–100% of patients with ongoing complete responses up until 7 years. The most common adverse events were local burning and soreness. Imiquimod is considered the treatment of choice for uVIN (Figures 19.9a and b).

(a)　　　　　　　　　　　　　　　　　　　(b)

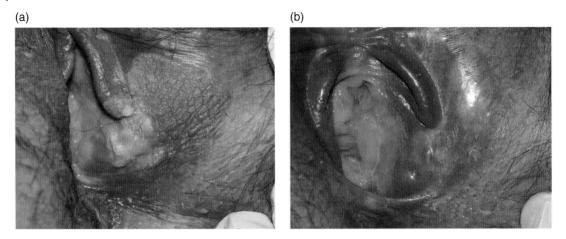

Figure 19.9 (a) Undifferentiated VIN and (b) after treatment with imiquimod.

Topical photodynamic therapy (PDT) uses a tumour-localizing photo sensitizer, 5-aminoevulinic acid (ALA), in combination with nonthermal light of an appropriate wavelength to generate oxygen-induced cell death. Photodynamic therapy has ablative and nonsurgical effects but has never been tested in a RCT in uVIN. It is well tolerated and has varying results. Again, the advantage over surgery is that, like imiquimod, it preserves the anatomy of the vulva.

Experimental therapeutic HPV vaccines have clinical responses and symptomatic improvement in nonrandomized studies in women with uVIN. Therapeutic vaccines have been developed to enhance T-cell mediated immunity in uVIN-lesions. Most vaccines cause specific immunity against the HPV E6 and E7 proteins. Therapeutic vaccination will play a role in the future in the treatment of uVIN, either alone or in combination with other modalities.

Cidofovir, a potent antiviral agent, when compared with imiquimod in a RCT, has been found to be equally effective in nearly 50% of patients.

A wait-and-see policy, aimed at controlling symptoms and prevention of malignancy, is an option in the management of uVIN in carefully selected patients. Frequent follow-up visits are advised, including careful examination and biopsies in cases of suspected malignancy.

In contrast, there is consensus on the best treatment of dVIN. This is surgical removal with a thorough pathological review to rule out a vulval SCC. No laser evaporization or any other ablative therapy, or immune modulation, should be used in these patients.

Progression

Although dVIN (Figures 19.10a and b) has a much higher malignant potential than uVIN (Figure 19.11), the malignant potential of uVIN should not be underestimated. In untreated uVIN up to 16% will develop vulval SCC within 8 years. The relatively short length of follow up may play a role in the underestimation of these figures. In treated patients, the rate of progression during follow up ranges from 2% to 6%. The progression rate is not affected by the extent of surgery. Free resection margins do not prevent progression to vulval SCC.

Therefore, one should not enlarge the extent of resection simply to prevent progression. In uVIN, occult vulval SCC can be found in nearly 20% in the excised specimen. This means that multiple

(a)

(b)

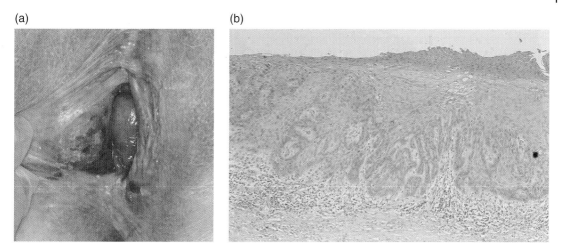

Figure 19.10 (a) Vulval SCC. (b) Labium majus, which developed in a region with dVIN on the background of LS.

Figure 19.11 Multifocal uVIN with progression to vulval SCC on the perineum.

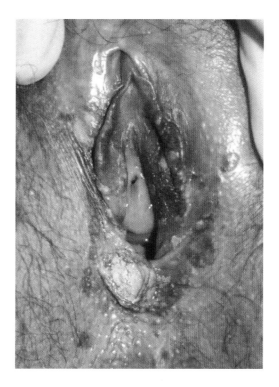

biopsies should be taken to rule out vulval SCC before a treatment plan is made. Known risk factors for progression of uVIN are related to advanced age, smoking, immunosuppression, previous radiotherapy in the lower genital tract, multifocality, large lesion size, raised lesions, positive surgical margins and basaloid type uVIN. There has been a small increase in the incidence of vulval SCC over the last 20 years and this is mainly due to an increase in younger women who tend to have a history of HPV infection and uVIN. The mean time to progression is nearly 5 years, but can occur after

18 years, indicating the importance of a long and careful follow up. Differentiated VIN lesions will progress to vulval SCC in less than 2 years in over 30%. The relation between a prior, synchronous or subsequent vulval carcinoma and dVIN is nearly 90% and three times higher than uVIN. Furthermore, vulval SCC arising on a background of dVIN is more likely to recur than one arising from uVIN. Overall, the prognosis is worse in patients with vulval SCC associated with dVIN than in patients with uVIN associated vulval SCC.

Melanoma *in situ*

Melanoma *in situ* (MIS) (Figure 19.12) is rare on the vulva and appears to have a relatively slow but definite progression to invasive melanoma. It is generally asymptomatic. All suspicious pigmented lesions on the vulva should be biopsied and a punch biopsy is the preferred method because establishing the depth of such lesions is critical. Destruction by cryosurgery,

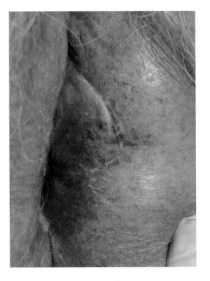

Figure 19.12 Vulval melanoma *in situ*.

cautery or laser is contraindicated and all such lesions must undergo careful histopathological evaluation. Small lesions can often be completely excised easily. When sampling hyperpigmented areas, a biopsy of the thickest region is recommended. Melanoma *in situ* should be excised with a margin of 5 mm of normal vulval skin.

When to Refer

Once uVIN, dVIN or MIS is diagnosed, the patient should be referred to a vulval specialist clinical with experience in treating these women.

Practice Points

- The two types of VIN, usual and differentiated, differ in prevalence, etiology, pathogenesis, histology, clinical presentation, and malignant potential.
- In patients with lichen sclerosus all lesions that do not respond to high potent steroid therapy should be biopsied to rule out dVIN or SCC.
- Differentiated VIN should be removed surgically.
- The usual type of VIN is related to persistent high-risk HPV infection with host inability to clear infection. In patients with multifocal pigmented, white or red lesions on the vulva uVIN should be suspected. A biopsy should be taken to confirm the clinical diagnosis.
- In patients with uVIN, other intraepithelial lesion in the lower genital tract should be looked for.
- In uVIN patients, multiple biopsies should be taken to rule out vulval squamous cell carcinoma before a treatment plan is made.
- Treatment of uVIN should be directed towards preservation of the anatomy and function of the vulva.
- The first-line treatment of uVIN is imiquimod.

Further Reading

Bornstein, J., Bogliatto, F., Haefner, H. K. *et al.* (2016) The 2015 International Society for the Study of Vulvo-vaginal Disease (ISSVD) terminology of vulvar squamous intraepithelial lesions. *Journal of Lower Genital Tract Disorders* **20**, 11–14.

De Vuyst, H., Clifford, G. M., Nascimento, M. C. *et al.* (2009) Prevalence and type distribution of human papillomavirus in carcinoma and intraepithelial neoplasia of the vulva, vagina and anus: a meta-analysis. *International Journal of Cancer* **124**, 1626–1636.

Iversen, T. and Tretli, S. (1998) Intraepithelial and invasive squamous cell neoplasia of the vulva: trends in incidence, recurrence, and survival rate in Norway. *Obstetrics and Gynecology* **91**, 969–972.

Jones, R. W., Rowan, D. M. and Stewart, A. W. (2005) Vulvar intraepithelial neoplasia. Aspects of the natural history and outcome in 405 women. *Obstetrics and Gynecology* **106**, 1319–1326.

Kaufman, R. H. (1995) Intraepithelial neoplasia of the vulva. *Gynecologic Oncology* **56**, 8–21.

Kaushik, S., Pepas, L., Nordin, A. *et al.* (2014) Surgical interventions for high-grade vulval intraepithelial neoplasia. *Cochrane Database of Systematic Reviews* **3** (Art. No.: CD007928). doi: 10.1002/14651858. CD007928.pub3

Nieuwenhof, van den H. P., Avoort, van der I. A., de Hullu, J. A. (2008) Review of squamous premalignant vulvar lesions. *Critical Reviews in Oncology/Hematology* **68**, 131–156.

Pepas, L., Kaushik, S., Nordin, A. *et al.* (2015) Medical interventions for high-grade vulval intraepithelial neoplasia. *Cochrane Database of Systematic Reviews* **8** (Art. No.: CD007924). doi: 10.1002/14651858. CD007924.pub3

Seters, M. van, Beurden, M. van, Craen, A. J. M. de. (2005) Is the assumed natural history of vulvar intraepithelial neoplasia III based on enough evidence? A systematic review of 3322 published patients. *Gynecologic Oncology* **97**, 545–551.

Seters, M. van, Beurden, M. van, ten Kate F. J. W., *et al.* (2008) Treatment of vulvar intraepithelial neoplasia with topical imiquimod. *New England Journal of Medicine* **358**, 1465–1473.

Sideri, M., Jones, R. W., Wilkinson, E. J. *et al.* (2005) Squamous vulvar intraepithelial neoplasia: 2004 modified terminology, ISSVD Vulvar Oncology Subcommittee. *Journal of Reproductive Medicine* **50**, 807–810.

Terlou, A., Blok, L. J., Helmerhorst, T. J. and van Beurden, M. (2010) Premalignant epithelial disorders of the vulva: squamous vulvar intraepithelial neoplasia, vulvar Paget's disease and melanoma in situ. *Acta Obstetricia et Gynecologica Scandinavica* **89**, 741–748.

Terlou, A., Seters, M. van, Ewing, P. C. *et al.* (2011) Treatment of vulvar intraepithelial neoplasia with topical imiquimod: seven years median follow-up of a randomized controlled trial. *Gynecologic Oncology* **121**, 157–162.

Useful Web Site for Patient Information

International Society for the Study of Vulvovaginal Disease:
http://www.issvd.org/3493/ (accessed 19 September 2016)

20

Extramammary Paget's Disease

Introduction

Vulval extramammary Paget's disease (EMPD) is a nonsquamous intraepithelial lesion of the vulva. It is an uncommon premalignant skin disorder with invasive potential. All areas that contain apocrine glands can be affected, such as the vulva, perianal region, penis, scrotum, perineum and axilla, but it most commonly occurs on the vulva. Extramammary Paget's disease of the vulva is defined by the presence of so-called Paget cells in the epithelium. Vulval EMPD spreads in an occult manner, often with more unseen lesions extending beyond the apparent edges. Vulval EMPD can be subclassified into primary or secondary disease. Primary disease originates on the vulva and secondary EMPD is due to a noncutaneous neoplasm, often of adjacent sites, such as the bladder or rectum. Interventions can be surgical, or noninvasive techniques may be applied. The purpose of the treatment is to remove the disease but also to reduce side effects from radical surgery. There is hardly any consensus on treatment.

Epidemiology

Even in a vulval clinic, EMPD is seen in less than 1% of the cases. It affects mainly white postmenopausal women, with a median age of 72 years. The true incidence and prevalence remains unknown. To date, only a couple of hundred cases are recorded in the literature. There is an uncertain association between vulval EMPD and distant tumours, such as those of the breast, pancreas, endometrium, bladder, stomach and rectum. The association is variable across the literature, ranging from 0–50%.

Histological Features

The histogenesis of primary vulval EMPD is still uncertain. There is evidence that vulval EMPD represents a heterogeneous group of epithelial neoplasms that can be similar both clinically and histopathologically. It has been speculated that it originates from eccrine and / or apocrine glands or from pluripotent keratinocyte cells of the epidermis or its adnexae. There is evidence that these glandular cells spread to the overlying epithelium. It has been suggested that at least a proportion of vulval EMPD arises multicentrically within the epidermis from these pluripotent stem cells. The diagnosis is histological with the characteristic changes on skin biopsy. Immunohistochemistry will help to exclude melanoma and vulval intraepithelial neoplasia as these are important histological

A Practical Guide to Vulval Disease: Diagnosis and Management, First Edition. Fiona Lewis, Fabrizio Bogliatto and Marc van Beurden.

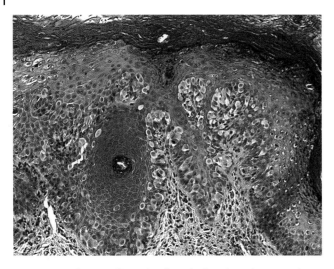

Figure 20.1 Clusters of Paget's cells with abundant clear cytoplasm and round nuclei in the basal layer.

differential diagnoses. Histopathology shows epidermal acanthosis and elongated rete ridges. Paget's cells are large intraepidermal cells with a large nucleus that often has a prominent nucleolus and abundant usually clear, mucin positive, pale cytoplasm. The cells may occur singly in small clusters or large nests (Figure 20.1). The squamous epithelium is often hyperplastic with hyper- or parakeratosis. The Paget's cells may extend into the adnexal duct and pilosebaceous units.

Classification

Vulval EMPD can be classified based on the origin of the neoplastic Paget's cells as either primary (of cutaneous origin), arising within the epithelium of the vulva, or secondary (of noncutaneous origin), resulting from the spread of an internal malignancy, most commonly from an anorectal adenocarcinoma or urothelial carcinoma of the bladder or urethra, to the vulval epithelium. The primary form comprises more than 75% of cases. Primary EMPD can be further subdivided into a primary, intraepithelial cutaneous form with and without invasion or an intraepithelial cutaneous Paget's disease as a manifestation of underlying skin appendage adenocarcinoma. Secondary EMPD has an anorectal, urothelial or other origin (Box 20.1).

These subtypes can present similarly on the skin and may appear similar on routine hematoxylin and eosin-stained slides. Immunohistochemical studies can be used to help differentiate them (Table 20.1). Primary vulval EMPD is immunoreactive for CK 7 and GCDFP-15 but uncommonly for CK 20. Vulval EMPD secondary to anorectal carcinoma demonstrates CK 20 immunoreactivity but is usually nonreactive for CK 7 and consistently nonimmunoreactive for GCDFP-15. Vulval EMPD secondary to urothelial carcinoma is immunoreactive for CK 7 and CK 20 but nonimmunoreactive for GCDFP-15. In addition, UP-III, which is specific for urothelium, is immunoreactive in secondary vulval EMPD of urothelial origin.

If vulval EMPD around the anus or urethra is present, look for tumours in the rectum or urethra.

Box 20.1 Classification of EMPD of the vulva (after Wilkinson and Brown, 2002).

Paget's disease of primary cutaneous Origin

- Primary intraepithelial neoplasm.
- Without invasion.
- With invasion.
- Manifestation of underlying skin appendage adenocarcinoma.

Paget's disease of noncutaneous origin

- Secondary to anorectal adenocarcinoma.
- Secondary to urothelial neoplasia.
- Manifestation of intraepithelial urothelial neoplasia.
- Manifestation of urothelial carcinoma.
- Secondary to another noncutaneous carcinoma (endocervical adenocarcinoma, endometrial adeno-carcinoma, ovarian carcinoma, etc.).

Table 20.1 Immunocytochemistry in EMPD.

	Primary EMPD	Secondary EMPD	Intraepithelial neoplasia	Melanoma
PAS	+	+	–	–
CK7	+	+	–	–
CK20	Usually –	Usually +	–	–
S100	–	–	–	+
Melan A	–	–	–	+

Symptoms

The most common symptoms are itching, burning, maceration and bleeding, sometimes for up to 5 years. Substantial delay between appearance of symptoms and diagnosis can occur in many patients.

Clinical Features

Vulval EMPD is usually asymmetrical, multifocal and may occur anywhere on the vulva, mons, peri-neum, perianal area or inner thigh (Figure 20.2). Vulval EMPD is characterized clinically as slowly expanding, often multiple extensive, sharply demarcated, moist, eczematoid lesions (Figure 20.3). These are erythematous or white patches and plaques but ulcers, nodules, focal hyperpigmentation and hypopigmentation can occur within them. Similar lesions can be seen perianally (Figure 20.4) and at this site a rectal or colonic malignancy should be looked for.

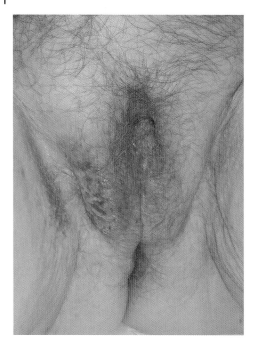

Figure 20.2 Extramammary Paget's disease affecting the right labium majus.

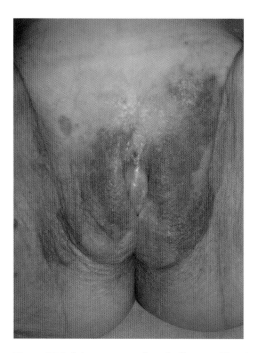

Figure 20.3 Extramammary Paget's disease with extensive sharply demarcated erythema with areas of hyperkeratosis, erosions and moist skin.

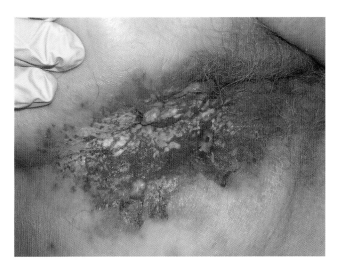

Figure 20.4 Extension of EMPD to the perianal area.

Management

Wide local excision is the usual treatment of vulval EMPD to a depth of 4–6 mm to include the pilosebaceous units and skin adnexal structures. It seems reasonable that surgery should be tailored to the size of the lesion. Alternative treatments are topical imiquimod (an immune response modifier), radiotherapy, chemotherapy, photodynamic therapy (topical and systemic) and laser therapy, or a combination of these approaches. There are no trials in the management of vulval EMPD. Patients with an underlying adnexal adenocarcinoma or stromal invasion of vulval EMPD over 1 mm should be treated more aggressively, with excision to the fascia in the involved area and bilateral inguinofemoral lymphadenectomy. Vulvoperineal reconstruction may be necessary by means of skin grafts, local skin flaps, muscle flaps and different fasciocutaneous flaps (see Figure 20.5). Surgical excision margins are often found to be positive. This is because subclinical EMPD is far more extensive on the vulva then the visible lesion. Therefore recurrences occur in up to 60% of cases. This leads to further surgery and the alteration of the normal vulval anatomy. Recurrences occur regardless of the histological status of the margins. There is no need to repeat surgery if the margins are positive, and thus it is not necessary to do intraoperative frozen sections. Surgical excision might mutilate the vulva with subsequent psychosexual morbidity.

Based on small series, topical 5% imiquimod cream has been shown as a safe treatment and may induce complete responses in primary or recurrent vulval EMPD. The therapeutic schedule used varies. A daily application for 3 weeks, followed by an every-other-day application for an additional 3 weeks seems to be effective.

Radiation therapy in selected cases may be feasible and may give good local control. This might be an alternative, particularly in medically inoperable patients. However, numbers as a first-line treatment are too small to draw any conclusions about disease-free and overall survival.

Targeted therapy with trastuzumab may be considered as a possible new therapeutic strategy in selected cases of vulval EMPD showing overexpression of HER-2/neu. Treatment can result in a significant regression of disease and resolution of symptoms. Chemotherapy is further given in metastatic adenocarcinoma. Mitomycin C, epirubicin, vincristin, cisplatin and 5-fluorouracil are used,

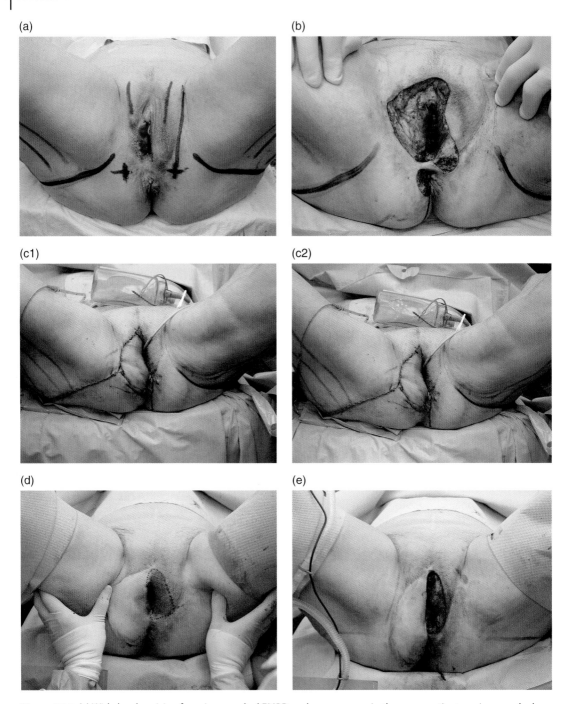

Figure 20.5 (a) Wide local excision for primary vulval EMPD and a recurrence in the same patient – primary vulval EMPD (courtesy of J. J. Hage, MD, PhD, plastic surgeon). (b) After the wide local excision. (c) Defect closed by fasciocutaneous infragluteal propeller flap. (d) Recurrence of vulval EMPD on the left side after 14 months' follow up. (e) Recurrence excised by wide local excision.

(f) 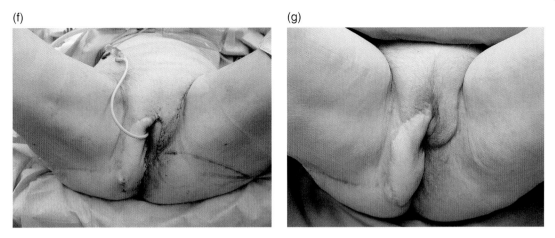 (g)

Figure 20.5 (Cont'd) (f) Defect closed by pedicled pudendal thigh island flap. (g) After 3 months' follow up.

but prognosis is poor in these cases. The role of photodynamic therapy in vulval EMPD is still unclear because only a few uncontrolled small series have been published with variable outcome and short follow up.

Laser therapy has only been applied in women with large, likely inoperable lesions with a high recurrence rate, so it is not possible to draw conclusions regarding the efficacy of the treatment.

Recurrences

Up to 60% of patients, treated by surgery will develop recurrences. This is related to the fact that the extent of histologically demonstrable disease is far greater than that of the visible lesion. The outline of the involved area is highly irregular and multiple foci of disease are present. Not surprisingly, the risk of recurrence appears to have a poor relationship with the status of the surgical margins. The extent of surgery, vulvectomy versus wide local excision, gives no difference in recurrence rate. Moh's surgery or the use of frozen sections do not improve surgical clearance or reduce recurrence rates. Local recurrences occur in half of the patients with tumour-free margins by frozen section and, conversely, if margins are involved, recurrences do not always appear.

Progression

Vulval EMPD is predominantly an intraepithelial lesion but it has the potential for dermal invasion and on occasions it has been associated with an underlying adenocarcinoma. Progression can occur more than 20 years after diagnosis. Associated vulval adenocarcinoma (4%) and invasive vulval EMPD (16%) may frequently coexist. Just as with the management of squamous cell carcinoma of the vulva, there is evidence to support the recognition of a category of minimally invasive vulval EMPD (less 1 mm depth of invasion) that has a low risk of distant metastasis and death caused by disease. These patients can be treated by surgical removal alone, whereas those with deeper invasion will need bilateral inguino-femoral lymphadenectomy.

Follow Up

Long-term monitoring is recommended, as recurrences are common and can be noted many years after the initial treatment. Repeat surgical excision is often necessary. Follow up is necessary to exclude both local recurrence and the development of associated internal malignancies. Follow up, at recommended intervals of 6–12 months is advised. Invasion is usually associated with symptoms. Once symptoms recur the patient should be further examined in between follow up visits.

When to Refer

Once EMPD is diagnosed, the patient should be referred to a vulval specialist clinical with experience in treating these women.

Practice Points

- A biopsy should be taken to confirm the clinical diagnosis.
- A CT scan of the abdomen and colonoscopy is advised in vulval EPMD. If EMPD around the anus or urethra is present, look for tumours in the rectum or urethra.
- In surgical treatment, histological radical removal is not necessary to prevent recurrence or progression.
- Imiquimod provides a viable alternative to surgical excision for vulval EMPD.
- Radiation therapy is a feasible alternative in medically inoperable patients.
- Long-term or lifelong follow up is recommended.

Further Reading

Edey, K. A., Allan, E., Murdoch, J. B. *et al.* (2013) Interventions for the treatment of Paget's disease of the vulva. *Cochrane Database of Systematic Reviews* **10** (Art. No.: CD009245). doi: 10.1002/14651858. CD009245.pub2

Fanning, J., Lambert, H. C., Hale, T. M. *et al.* (1999) Paget's disease of the vulva: prevalence of associated vulval adenocarcinoma, invasive Paget's disease, and recurrence after surgical excision. *American Journal of Obstetrics and Gynecology* **180**, 24–27.

Gunn, R. A. and Gallager, H. S. (1980) Vulval Paget's disease. A topographic study. *Cancer* **46**, 590–594.

Hage, J. J. and van Beurden, M. (2011) Reconstruction of acquired perineovulval defects: A proposal of sequence. *Seminars in Plastic Surgery* **25**, 148–154.

Machida, H., Moeini, A., Roman, L. D. and Matsuo, K. (2015) Effects of imiquimod on vulval Paget's disease: A systematic review of literature. *Gynecologic Oncology* **139**, 165–171.

MacLean, A. B., Makwana, M., Ellis, E. P. and Cunnington, F. (2004) The management of Paget's disease of the vulva. Review. *Journal of Obstetrics and Gynaecology* **24**, 124–128.

Regauer, S. (2006) Extramammary Paget's disease – a proliferation of adnexal origin? *Histopathology* **48**, 723–729.

Terlou, A., Blok, L. J., Helmerhorst, T. J. and van Beurden, M. (2010) Premalignant epithelial disorders of the vulva: squamous vulval intraepithelial neoplasia, vulval Paget's disease and melanoma in situ. *Acta Obstetricia et Gynecologica Scandinavica* **89**, 741–748.

Wilkinson, R. J. and Brown, H. (2002) Vulval Paget disease of urothelial origin: a report of three cases and a proposed classification of vulval Paget disease. *Human Pathology* **33**, 549–554.

Yamazaki, N., Yamamoto, A., Wada, T. *et al.* (1999) A case of metastatic extramammary Paget's disease that responded to combination chemotherapy. *Journal of Dermatology* **26**, 311–316.

Useful Web Site for Patient Information

International Society for the Study of Vulvovaginal Disease:
http://www.issvd.org/extra-mammary-pagets-disease/ (accessed 19 September 2016)

21

Vulval Squamous Cell Carcinoma

Introduction

Vulval cancer accounts for approximately 4% of all gynaecological malignancies and 1% of all cancers in women. Ninety per cent of vulval cancer consists of squamous cell carcinoma. Vulval squamous cell carcinoma (VSCC) is the fourth most common gynaecologic cancer, following cancer of the uterine corpus, ovary and cervix. The five-year survival rate is 70% but morbidity is high, despite the change in surgery to less invasive procedures over the last few decades, which has not changed survival but has decreased the complication rate and improved quality of life. This is particularly important because the rate of vulval cancer in younger women has increased dramatically since the 1960s due to the rise in HPV-related tumours.

Epidemiology

Vulval squamous cell carcinoma is mainly diagnosed in elderly women with a mean age at diagnosis of approximately 70 years. Fifteen per cent occur in women under 50 years of age. The incidence is around 2 per 100 000 women per year. Mortality rates have been stable in younger women but have declined in older women. Risk factors are HPV-related undifferentiated vulval intraepithelial neoplasia (uVIN) and lichen sclerosis (LS). Risk factors associated with HPV infection include early age at first intercourse, multiple sexual partners, human immunodeficiency virus (HIV) infection and cigarette smoking.

Aetiology / Histology

Two independent pathways of vulvar carcinogenesis currently exist, both with their own premalignant lesions and invasive histologic forms. One type is related to LS and the second type is related to HPV infection. The most common type occurs in elderly women on a background of LS and often differentiated VIN (dVIN) and leads to mostly keratinizing carcinoma. There is no relation to HPV. Differentiated VIN is underreported and has probably a relatively short intraepithelial phase before progression starts (see Chapter 19). The second type consists of mainly nonkeratinizing carcinomas and affects primarily younger women. It is caused predominantly by HPV 16 and 18 infection, resulting in undiffentiated VIN (uVIN), which may lead to VSCC. These women tend to present with early-stage disease.

Verrucous carcinoma is a variant of VSCC with cauliflower-like appearance (Figure 21.1). It has a verrucous configuration on histology. The lesion grows slowly and rarely metastasizes to lymph nodes but it may be locally destructive.

A Practical Guide to Vulval Disease: Diagnosis and Management, First Edition. Fiona Lewis, Fabrizio Bogliatto and Marc van Beurden.
© 2017 John Wiley & Sons Ltd. Published 2017 by John Wiley & Sons Ltd.

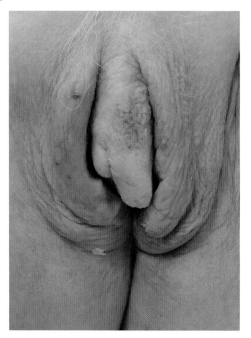

Figure 21.1 Verrucous squamous cell carcinoma.

Symptoms and Clinical Features

Pruritus or pain is a common complaint. Vulval bleeding or discharge, dysuria, or an enlarged lymph node in the groin, are less frequently encountered symptoms and suggestive of advanced disease. On the other hand, patients may be asymptomatic at the time of diagnosis. Most patients present with a unifocal vulval plaque, ulcer or mass on either the background of multifocal uVIN or LS. Multifocality may be present. A synchronous second malignancy, most commonly cervical neoplasia, is found in up to 20% of patients.

Vulval squamous cell carcinoma metastasizes by a variety of mechanisms. Modes of spread include direct extension to adjacent structures (e.g. vagina, urethra, clitoris, anus), lymphatic spread to regional lymph nodes and hematogenous dissemination. Most VSCC spread first to the groin, which is why these nodes are sampled as part of staging (see Box 21.1). Lymphatic spread to regional lymph nodes can occur early in the course of disease, even in patients with small lesions. Lesions that are on one side of the vulva generally spread only to the ipsilateral groin nodes. The pretreatment risk of groin lymph node metastases appears to be in the order of 15%. Lymphatic spread does not occur in lesions with less than 1 mm depth of invasion. In tumours up to 2 mm, the chance of invasion is 8%, and in those more than 5 mm, 34% are likely to have lymph node involvement. Groin lymph node metastases are associated with a poorer prognosis and adjuvant radiotherapy is indicated in these patients. Palpation of the groin is part of the physical examination but this it inadequate. Among patients with no enlargement with palpation of groin nodes, 16% to 24% have clinically occult metastases. Hematogenous dissemination, which typically occurs late in the course of the disease to lungs, liver and bones, is rare in patients without inguinofemoral lymph-node involvement.

Management

If a benign vulvar lesion is initially suspected, but does not respond to common treatment, biopsy is recommended to exclude malignancy and establish a diagnosis. All abnormal skin lesions should be individually biopsied to 'map' all potential sites of vulvar pathology as VSCC may be seen in areas with multifocal uVIN.

Surgery

Historically, the rate of surgical complications following VSCC was high, occurring in up to 85% of patients and resulting in a significant decrease of quality of life (QOL). In recent decades, treatment has become less radical. Routine pelvic lymphadenectomy was omitted. Wide local excision

---

Box 21.1 FIGO staging of vulval cancer.

  1) Tumour confined to the vulva.
 1a) Lesions ≤2 cm in size, confined to the vulva or perineum and with stromal invasion ≤1.0 mm.
 1b) Lesions >2 cm in size with stromal invasion >1.0 mm, confined to the vulva or perineum.
  2) Tumour of any size with extension to adjacent perineal structures (lower/distal 1/3 urethra, lower/distal 1/3 vagina, anal involvement).
  3) Tumour of any size with or without extension to adjacent perineal structures (lower/distal 1/3 urethra, lower/distal 1/3 vagina, anal involvement) with positive inguino-femoral lymph nodes.
 4a) Tumour of any size with extension to any of the following: upper/proximal 2/3 of urethra, upper/proximal 2/3 vagina, bladder mucosa, rectal mucosa, or fixed to pelvic bone.
 4b) Any distant metastases including pelvic lymph nodes.

---

became the standard instead of vulvectomy for patients with unifocal tumours. For microinvasive tumours with less then ≤1 mm invasion and with a maximum diameter of ≤2 cm (FIGO 1a), patients are treated with a wide local excision only and treatment of the groin can be safely omitted because lymph node metastases are extremely rare in this group. This is in contrast to tumours with >1 mm invasion, which have a risk of nodal metastases of up to 34%. The use of separate groin incisions for the inguinal-femoral lymphadenectomy instead of *en bloc* resection improved wound healing dramatically without compromising survival. A sentinel node (SN) procedure in patients with a unifocal tumour <4 cm without abnormal groin nodes is safe and results in less than 2.5% groin recurrences after long-term follow up. Treatment-related morbidity is minimal. Therefore SN dissection should be part of the standard treatment in selected patients with early stage vulval cancer.

Surgical margins should be 1–2 cm, decreasing the chance of local recurrences. Dissection should go down to the deep fascia and to the periosteum of the pubic symphysis. Reconstructive surgery is often necessary to prevent wound complications (Figure 21.2) but psychosexual sequelae might not be prevented completely by these operations. If the margins on histology are ≤8 mm, there is a high risk of local recurrences. Unilateral rather than bilateral lymphadenectomy is performed whenever possible because it decreases postoperative morbidity. In lateral disease unilateral lymphadenectomy is associated with a <3% risk of contralateral groin node metastases. A unilateral lymphadenectomy is recommended for women with a lesion >1 cm from the vulvar midline and no palpable groin nodes on examination or abnormal lymph nodes on ultrasound. Vulval squamous cell carcinoma often coexist with premalignant uVIN or dVIN. At the time of surgical treatment, intraepithelial neoplasia should be excised but it is not necessary to excise benign lesions, such as LS.

These developments in surgical treatment led to improved recovery, shorter hospital stays, less psychosexual dysfunction and a reduction in morbidity. Despite these changes, morbidity following surgery to the vulva and groins is still significant.

Complications

Treatment is still associated with significant physical, sexual, and psychological morbidity. Complications are lymphedema, lymphocele formation, wound complications, cellulitis, pelvic floor prolapse, urinary or stool incontinence and rarely necrotizing fasciitis and osteomyelitis pubis.

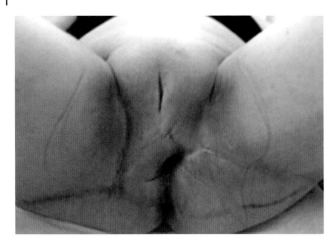

Figure 21.2 Plastic reconstruction is often necessary to prevent wound complications. Psychosexual sequalae might still be significant (courtesy of J. J. Hage, MD, PhD, plastic surgeon).

Lymphedema occurs in up to 50% of patients after inguinal-femoral lymphadenectomy. There have been complaints of leg swelling or heaviness of the lower limbs, typically within 12 months of treatment. Once developed, this often becomes chronic. There are several risk factors, such as obesity, number of lymph nodes removed, extent of surgery, postoperative infection and radiation therapy to the groin, which increase the risk of developing lymphedema after inguinal-femoral lymphadenectomy. The most effective means of preventing lymphedema is by omitting the inguinal-femoral lymphadenectomy. This can be achieved safely through the SN procedure. Leg lymphedema will occur in less than 2% after a SN procedure.

Lymphocele formation is noted in up to 40% of patients after inguinal-femoral lymphadenectomy. Often this is self-limiting but sometimes repeated drainage is necessary.

Wound complications are common and a serious cause of morbidity in patients undergoing surgical treatment for VSCC. Up to 60% of patients undergoing vulvectomy suffer wound complications following surgery. Wound complications have decreased dramatically since the implementation of separate groin incisions. Risk factors are obesity, diabetes mellitus and extent of the procedure. The SN procedure also dramatically lowers the risk for wound complications compared to inguinal-femoral lymphadenectomy. There is very limited evidence concerning the use of drains and rate of complications following surgery to the groin in patients with VSCC.

Sexual dysfunction and psychosocial issues are reported in over half of the women and have enormous impact on a patient's quality of life. The extreme changes to the anatomy of the vulva can result in dyspareunia, negative feelings about body image, decreased desire and inability to orgasm. Many women therefore abandon sex completely after vulvectomy.

Radiotherapy

For women with two or more microscopically positive groin lymph nodes, one or more macroscopically involved lymph nodes, or any evidence of extracapsular spread, adjuvant radiation therapy (RT) is indicated. Primary radiotherapy to the groin results in less morbidity, especially lymphedema, but may be associated with a higher risk of groin recurrence and decreased survival when compared with surgery. Surgery should still be considered the first-line treatment for the groin nodes in women with

VSCC. If the condition of the patient gives an increased risk of morbidity with the use of surgery, then primary radiotherapy is a good alternative treatment. For patients who have tumours that might not be technically resectable, chemoradiation is appropriate in patients with ano-rectal, urethral, or bladder involvement in an effort to avoid colostomy and urostomy, lymphangitis cutis, disease that is fixed to the bone and possibly immobile or ulcerative inguinal-femoral lymph node involvement. Chemotherapy given is cisplatin, mitomycin-C or 5-FU.

Follow Up

Local recurrence rate after primary treatment and after long-term follow up is as high as 40%. Lifetime observation is therefore necessary. Follow up, at recommended intervals of 6–12 months, is advised. Recurrence is usually associated with symptoms. Once symptoms recur, the patient should be further examined in between follow up visits.

Prognosis

Inguinal-femoral lymph node involvement is the most significant prognostic factor for survival in patients with vulvar cancer. Fiveyear survival ranges from 70 to 93% for patients with negative nodes, to 25 to 41% for those with positive nodes. Other prognostic factors include stage, capillary lymphatic space invasion and older age. Survival rates for FIGO stage 1–4 are 79%, 59%, 43% and 13% respectively. Outcomes seem to improve over time, although surgical procedures became less aggressive, which may be attributable to advances in adjuvant therapy and more younger patients with less advanced disease at presentation.

When to Refer

Once VSCC is diagnosed the patient should be referred to a gynaecology oncology centre that specializes in treating these women.

Practice Points

- A benign lesion of the vulva that does not respond to standard treatment should be biopsied.
- If multiple abnormal areas are present in a patient with VSCC then multiple biopsies should be taken to 'map' all potential sites of vulvar pathology.
- Women with FIGO stage 1a VSCC require surgical resection of the primary lesion alone without inguinal-femoral lymphadenectomy.
- A sentinel node (SN) procedure in patients with a unifocal tumour <4 cm without abnormal groin nodes is safe and results in less than 2.5% groin recurrences after long-term follow up and treatment-related morbidity is minimal.
- Surgical margins should be 1–2 cm to prevent local recurrences.
- For women with lateral lesions <4 cm without abnormal lymph nodes a unilateral lymphadenectomy is appropriate.

- For women with two or more microscopically positive groin lymph nodes, one or more macroscopically involved lymph nodes, or any evidence of extracapsular spread, adjuvant radiation therapy (RT) is indicated.
- Primary chemoradiation is feasible for patients with irresectable tumours.
- Radiation therapy is a feasible alternative in medically inoperable patients.
- Lifelong follow up is recommended.

Further Reading

Covens, A., Vella, E. T., Kennedy, E. B. *et al.* (2015) Sentinel lymph node biopsy in vulvar cancer: Systematic review, meta-analysis and guideline recommendations. *Gynecologic Oncology* **137**, 351–361.

De Hullu, J. A., Hollema, H., Lolkema, S. *et al.* (2002) Vulvar carcinoma. The price of less radical surgery. *Cancer* **95**, 2331.

FIGO Committee on Gynecologic Oncology (2014) FIGO staging for carcinoma of the vulva, cervix, and corpus uteri. *International Journal of Gynecology and Obstetrics* **125**, 97–98.

Knol, A. C. and Hage, J. J. (1997) The infragluteal skin flap: A new option for reconstruction in the perineogenital area. *Plastic and Reconstructive Surgery* **99**, 1954–1959.

Lawrie, T. A., Patel, A., Martin-Hirsch, P. P. L. *et al.* (2014) Sentinel node assessment for diagnosis of groin lymph node involvement in vulval cancer. *Cochrane Database of Systematic Reviews* **6** (Art. No.: CD010409). doi: 10.1002/14651858.CD010409.pub2

Micheletti, L. and Preti, M. (2014) Surgery of the vulva in vulvar cancer. *Best Practice and Research: Clinical Obstetrics and Gynaecology* **28**, 1074–1087.

te Grootenhuis, N. C., van der Zee, A. G. J., van Doorn, H. C. *et al.* (2016) Sentinel nodes in vulvar cancer: Long-term follow-up of the GROningen INternational Study on Sentinel nodes in Vulvar cancer (GROINSS-V) I. *Gynecologic Oncology* **140**, 8–14.

van der Velden, J., Fons, G. and Lawrie, T. A. (2011) Primary groin irradiation versus primary groin surgery for early vulvar cancer. *Cochrane Database of Systematic Reviews* **5** (Art. No.: CD002224). doi: 10.1002/14651858.CD002224.pub2.

Van der Zee, A. G. J., Oonk, M. H., De Hullu, J. A. *et al.* (2008) Sentinel node dissection is safe in the treatment of early-stage vulvar cancer. *Journal of Clinical Oncology* **26**, 884–889.

Wills, A. and Obermair, A. (2013) A review of complications associated with the surgical treatment of vulvar cancer. *Gynecologic Oncology* **131**(2), 467–479.

Useful Web Site for Patient Information

International Society for the Study of Vulvovaginal Disease:
http://www.issvd.org/vulvar-cancer/ (accessed 19 September 2016)

22

Other Vulval Cancers

The most common vulval cancer is a squamous cell carcinoma (see Chapter 21). The other important cancers that can affect the vulva are basal cell carcinoma and melanoma, which will be discussed in this chapter.

Basal Cell Carcinoma

Basal cell carcinoma (BCC) is the commonest malignant tumour to affect humans, and accounts for over 75% of skin cancers. There is a significant association with chronic sun exposure and, hence, 90% of these tumours are found on sun-exposed sites such as the head and neck or backs of hands.

Epidemiology

Vulval BCC is rare with approximately 300 cases reported in the literature. They are most common in Caucasians over the age of 60.

Incidence

Vulval basal cell carcinoma accounts for 2–4% of all vulval cancers and for less than 1% of BCCs overall.

Pathophysiology

As the vulva is a sun-protected site, sun exposure cannot be implicated as an aetiological factor. Chronic irritation, friction and human papilloma virus infection have been postulated but not proven.

Histological Features

The histological features of vulval BCC are identical to those found elsewhere. Invasive nests of cells bud off from the basal epithelium with characteristic palisading of the nuclei at the periphery. Some may show squamous differentiation.

It is possible to confuse BCC with the basaloid form of squamous vulval intraepithelial neoplasia. The BerEP4 stain may be helpful as this is generally positive in BCC.

A Practical Guide to Vulval Disease: Diagnosis and Management, First Edition. Fiona Lewis, Fabrizio Bogliatto and Marc van Beurden.
© 2017 John Wiley & Sons Ltd. Published 2017 by John Wiley & Sons Ltd.

Symptoms

Pruritus is reported but the lesions may be an incidental finding with the patient noticing a lump. Pain can occur, especially if there is clitoral involvement.

Clinical Features

The classic features seen in BCC are a pearly papule with surface telangiectasia (Figure 22.1). The centre may eventually ulcerate, giving rise to the term 'rodent ulcer'. On the vulva, this appearance is not always obvious and the lesion may be an erythematous papule or plaque (Figure 22.2), with or without ulceration. Vulval BCCs are frequently pigmented. They are most commonly found on the outer labia, mons and lower buttocks but have been reported on the inner labia, fourchette and clitoris. The major clinical differential diagnoses are of extramammary Paget's, benign lesions or mucous cysts.

As at other sites, the lesions usually grow slowly and may be present for many years before diagnosis. They are rarely aggressive but isolated reports of metastases to the inguinal nodes exist.

Basic Management

The management is surgical excision but local recurrence has been reported in up to 20% of vulval BCCs. Moh's micrographic surgery is the treatment of choice. Simple destructive procedures such as curettage, which are often used at other sites, are not so effective on the vulva, especially on hair-bearing areas and the lesions frequently recur. The same is true for imiquimod.

When to Refer

- Refer for consideration of Moh's micrographic surgery.
- Any recurrent lesion.

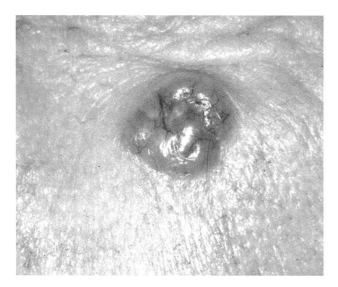

Figure 22.1 Typical appearances of BCC – pearly papule.

Figure 22.2 Vulval BCC – small nodule on outer labium majus.

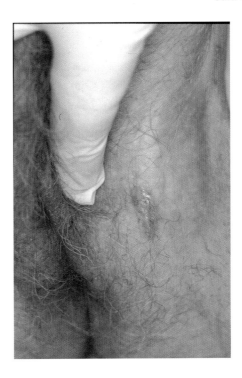

Practice Points

- Consider a BCC in all atypical papules or small ulcerated lesions and biopsy early.
- Follow-up for any signs of recurrence.
- Perform full skin examination to exclude lesions elsewhere.

Further Reading

De Giorgi, V., Salvini, C., Massi, D. *et al.* (2005) Vulvar BCC: retrospective study and review of the literature. *Gynecologic Oncology* **97**, 192–194.

Useful Web Site for Patient Information

British Association for Dermatologists:
http://www.bad.org.uk/library-media/documents/Basal%20Cell%20Carcinoma%20Update%20Feb%202012%20-%20lay%20reviewed%20Dec%202011(3).pdf (accessed 14 September 2016)

Malignant Melanoma

Melanoma of the vulva is rare but is the second most common vulval cancer, accounting for up to 10% of vulval malignant tumours. It is an aggressive disease with a poorer prognosis than at other sites.

Epidemiology

The average age at presentation is 60 and over 85% of the patients who develop a vulval melanoma are Caucasian. There are no known aetiologial factors for vulval melanoma as sun exposure is not relevant at this site.

Pathophysiology

Recent work has focused on genetic mutations in melanoma. The BRAF mutation is the most common cutaneous melanoma but in mucosal lesions, including those on the vulva, C-KIT and NRAS mutations are more frequent. There are now several inhibitors available as therapeutic options for these patients and so establishing the mutation for an individual patient is important in planning treatment.

As expected, a poorer prognosis correlates to a greater Breslow thickness, ulceration and the presence of lymph-node involvement.

Histological Features

A melanoma shows asymmetry and is poorly circumscribed. There is significant cytological atypia and nests of abnormal melanocytes of varying shape and size. Higher numbers of mitotic figures and the presence of ulceration are poor prognostic factors.

Symptoms

Early lesions are usually asymptomatic and as the site is not easily visible, diagnosis is often made late. If the lesion is nodular, then the patient may notice a lump and if it ulcerates, it may become painful.

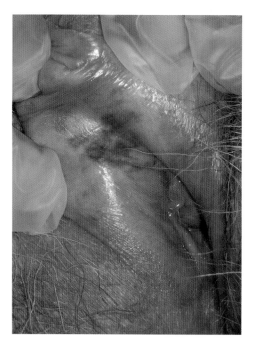

Figure 22.3 Melanoma right labium minus.

Clinical Features

Lesions may be macular, nodular or polypoidal. The inner labia minora and clitoris are most commonly affected (Figure 22.3) but the lesions are frequently multifocal and can be extensive at diagnosis (Figure 22.4). They will often have variations in colour, with brown, black and red areas (Figure 22.5). Vulval melanoma commonly exhibit amelanotic components.

Basic Management

Patients should be treated in specialist centres with access to a multidisciplinary team that includes dermatologists, gynaecologists, oncologists, expert nursing and palliative care specialists. Individualized management based on mutation of the tumour is now possible.

Patients will require imaging (CT/PET scanning) to determine the extent of disease and to establish any distant metastatic spread. Surgical excision is the mainstay of treatment with wide local excision and sentinel lymph-node biopsy generally offered.

Figure 22.4 Extensive nodular malignant melanoma.

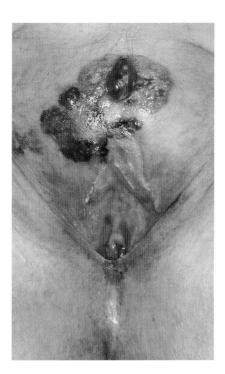

Figure 22.5 Variation in colour with amelanotic areas.

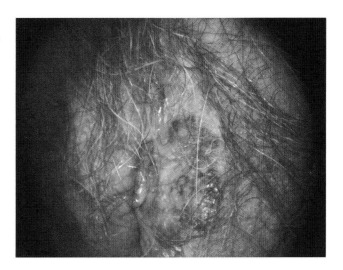

Further Reading

Janco, J. M. T., Markovic, S. N., Weaver, A. L. and Cliby, W. A. (2013) Vulvar and vaginal melanoma: Case series and review of current management options including neoadjuvant chemotherapy. *Gynaecologic Oncology* **129**, 533–537.

Rouzbahman, M., Kamel-Reid, S., Al Habeeb, A. *et al.* (2015) Malignant melanoma of vulva and vagina: a histomorphological review and meta analysis – a single centre study. *Journal of Lower Genital Tract Disorders* **19**, 350–353.

Tcheung, W. J., Selim, M. A., Herndon, J. E. *et al.* (2012) Clinicopathological study of 85 cases of melanoma of the female genitalia. *Journal of the American Academy of Dermatology* **67**, 598–605.

Wechter, M. E., Gruber, S. B., Haefner, H. K. *et al.* (2004) Vulvar melanoma: a report of 20 cases and review of the literature. *Journal of the American Academy of Dermatology* **50**, 554–562.

Other Malignant Tumours and the Vulva

Other soft tissue tumours can affect the vulva but are uncommon. Metastatic carcinoma can occur on the vulva, most commonly from the uterine cervix. The prognosis is extremely poor. Any atypical lesion should be biopsied to establish the diagnosis and the patient referred to a specialist clinic for further management.

Further Reading

Calonje, E. and Spiegel, G. W. (2009) Non-epithelial tumours of the vulva, in *Ridley's The Vulva*, 3rd edn (eds S. M. Neill and F. M. Lewis). Wiley-Blackwell, London, pp. 199–220.

23

Vulvodynia

Definition

The term ***vulvodynia*** was introduced for the first time in 1983 by the International Society for the Study of Vulvovaginal Disease. It was then subjected to discussion and reassessment, which led to a more precise definition, agreed in 2003. It was then defined as 'vulval pain in the absence of relevant, visible physical findings, or a specific clinically identifiable neurological disorder'.

This definition clearly introduces the concept that vulval pain due to specific diseases (such as herpes, or lichen sclerosus) must not be defined using the term vulvodynia. This term identifies a neuropathic pain, due to a dysfunction in peripheral and central nervous system pain processing. In this sense, vulvodynia is a type of allodynia, a term used to describe pain caused by a stimulus that in normal conditions does not provoke pain. Vulvodynia is not a symptom but a chronic pain syndrome where pain becomes a true disease.

In view of this, a review of the classification was agreed in 2015 (see Box 23.1). This now relates to 'persistent vulval pain' including such pain caused by a specific disorder. It also lists common comorbidities seen in these women.

Two specific subsets of vulvodynia, based on clinical features, have emerged (Figure 23.1). There are patients who describe constant generalized pain and those who have more localized pain that is provoked by touch or pressure. This latter group was described previously as having 'vestibulitis'. The 2003 classification suggested that the suffix *-itis* should no longer be used as this implies that inflammation is the main pathogenic element in this type of vulval pain. The term ***vestibulodynia*** is now used for this localized pain at the vestibule. There may be some overlap with spontaneous and provoked types occurring in the same patient.

Epidemiology

Vulvodynia has been estimated to affect up to 16% of women at some time. It can occur in all age groups and ethnicities. Localized provoked pain tends to occur in younger women and is most common in the 20–40 year age group.

A Practical Guide to Vulval Disease: Diagnosis and Management, First Edition. Fiona Lewis, Fabrizio Bogliatto and Marc van Beurden.
© 2017 John Wiley & Sons Ltd. Published 2017 by John Wiley & Sons Ltd.

Box 23.1 2015 consensus terminology and classification of persistent vulval pain.

A. Vulval pain caused by a specific disorder*

- Infectious (e.g. recurrent candidiasis, herpes)
- Inflammatory (e.g. lichen sclerosus, lichen planus, immunobullous disorders)
- Neoplastic (e.g. Paget disease, squamous cell carcinoma)
- Neurologic (e.g. postherpetic neuralgia, nerve compression or injury, neuroma)
- Trauma (e.g. female genital cutting, obstetrical)
- Iatrogenic (e.g. postoperative, chemotherapy, radiation)
- Hormonal deficiencies (e.g. genito-urinary syndrome of menopause (vulvo-vaginal atrophy), lactational amenorrhea)

B. Vulvodynia – Vulval pain of at least 3 months duration, without clear identifiable cause, which may have potential associated factors

Descriptors:

- Localized (e.g. vestibulodynia, clitorodynia) or generalized or mixed (localized and generalized)
  - Provoked (e.g. insertional, contact) or spontaneous or mixed (provoked and spontaneous)
  - Onset (primary or secondary)
- Temporal pattern (intermittent, persistent, constant, immediate, delayed)

Potential factors associated with vulvodynia

- Comorbidities and other pain syndromes (e.g. painful bladder syndrome, fibromyalgia, irritable bowel syndrome, temporomandibular disorder)
- Genetics
- Hormonal factors (e.g. pharmacologically induced)
- Inflammation
- Musculoskeletal (e.g. pelvic muscle overactivity, myofascial, biomechanical)
- Neurologic mechanisms: central, peripheral, neuroproliferative
- Psychosocial factors (e.g. mood, interpersonal, coping, role, sexual function)
- Structural defects (e.g. perineal descent)

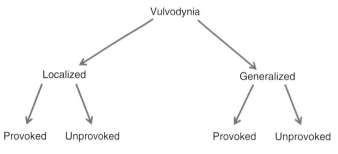

Figure 23.1 Subsets of vulvodynia.

Pathophysiology

The pathogenesis of vulvodynia is complex and multifactorial. Initially, inflammation was considered a significant factor in the onset and exacerbation of disease and a lot of attention was given to it. With the identification of neuropathic processes, the role of inflammation has been disproved, underlining the ISSVD recommendation to abandon the term 'vestibulitis'. Over the years several other factors were postulated such as infection (HPV, Candida, HSV), oxalate secretion in urine, modification of the microbial ecosystem of the vulva, altered sensory perception, peripheral neuropathy, an abnormality in the muscular tone of the pelvic floor, iatrogenic, hormonal and psychological factors. None of these is believed to be a significant aetiological factor.

It is now considered that the pathogenesis is that of neuropathic pain, which may be triggered or modified by psychological situations (sorrow, neglect, anxiety) or pathological states such as recurrent infections, increased muscular tone, perineal trauma. There is an increased frequency of other conditions with similar pain pathology – for example, fibromyalgia, irritable bladder, irritable bowel syndrome, migraine, facial pain and chronic fatigue syndrome.

Psychological Aspects of Vulvodynia

Sexual and psychological effects are common in these patients. They can develop severe problems with relationships because of their disease and it can be questioned that vulvodynia may be the 'lesser evil' that protects them from deeper psychological distresses. There is a higher incidence of anxiety in these patients but this is thought to be secondary to the chronic symptoms.

Some authors have suggested that vulvodynia should be considered as a functional disorder symptom or a somatization. The tendency to use the body to communicate psychological distress to the point of producing symptoms or organic diseases has been well known for years. This has to be differentiated from the simple somatic symptoms that occur due to stress. It is clear that under pressure some organic functions can be compromised but it is less clear why the altered function persists once the stress is over, or why the somatic symptom would involve different organs. The choice of the vulva as an area of somatization expression is a mystery but it has serious consequences because it prevents a normal sex life and often compromises social relationships.

The medical history of a woman with vulvodynia should include some information regarding her sexuality as a correct sexual history will be helpful to the therapeutic strategy. For instance, vulvodynia can be an expression of deep psychological conflicts such as hidden gender identity issues or homosexual feelings. Any possible conflict between partners should be evaluated. Feelings of anger associated with intercourse, fury at being a woman, feelings of victimization or negative feelings towards the partner should be explored. The reaction of the partner to her symptoms can have a significant impact on the outcome and feelings of anger expressed by the partner can reinforce her maladaptive behaviour to the problem.

Some aspects of sexual relationships are learned from personal experience observed in family members. A history of abuse in other close relatives can be relevant and may not be reported by the patient. However, there is no evidence that there is an increased incidence of physical or sexual abuse in patients with vulvodynia.

Vulvodynia may also have an effect on social functioning. If normal psychosexual development does not occur and there is a misrepresentation of sexuality, this can lead to preconceptions that vulval pain shows sexual incompetence. The trivialization of sexuality in the media, without taking into account the emotional factors involved, can have an impact on any vulval symptoms.

Histology

Histology has no diagnostic role and is not helpful. A mild, nonspecific lymph-histiocytic infiltrate was demonstrated in patients affected by vestibule pain and vulvodynia. However, more recent studies show that an inflammatory infiltrate is not correlated with clinical features as it is seen in asymptomatic women as well. Increased vestibular innervation is seen but the demonstration of nerve fibre proliferation does not necessarily imply pathology as this is related to the sensitivity to stimuli. Immuno-histochemical techniques are not able to differentiate afferent fibres from nociceptors (pain conductors) or proprioceptors (pressure conductors).

Symptoms

The onset of the symptoms may be gradual or sudden. There is frequently an initiating event that precedes the pain. This is commonly an episode of infection such as a urinary tract infection or candidiasis. This is treated appropriately but the symptoms of pain do not resolve. Patients often describe the pain in terms of burning, rawness, soreness, pricking or knifelike. Itch is not a feature. Pain may be felt over the whole vulva or localized to specific areas, most commonly the vestibule or clitoris. The pain can be spontaneous and occur randomly or constantly in the absence of any physical stimulus. This may spread to the thighs or perianal area.

The more common type is pain that is provoked by a stimulus such as touch or pressure as with sexual contact or tampon insertion. Patients may also find that their symptoms are provoked by wearing tight clothing, cycling or horse riding. In clinical practice, the posterior vestibule is the commonest site of localized provoked pain (vestibulodynia). Both types of vulvodynia are often associated with vaginismus and, as a consequence, sexual penetrative activity may become impossible. In generalized spontaneous vulvodynia, intercourse is possible but may be painful but in vestibulodynia it is often impossible due to the pain and secondary vaginismus. Patients with vaginismus show vestibular hyperreflexia to any touch stimulus and therefore develop muscular activity at minimum levels of stimulation. This situation is not restricted to vulvodynia but the prolonged contraction of the pubo-coccygeus muscle can cause myalgia.

Signs

Inspection of the vulva is normal in vulvodynia. It is important to search for any signs of infective or inflammatory disease. There should not be any relevant findings to explain the symptoms. For example, a wart or angiokeratoma may be seen but this would not explain widespread burning pain. The diagnostic test for vestibulodynia is the cotton-swab touch test. A cotton swab is used to give a light touch on the vestibule to map the distribution of hypersensitivity and pain.

In some cases, the delicate introduction of a speculum can be used to establish the presence of introital pain and to check for any discharge or other potential cause of the symptoms. Neurological examination is normal.

Investigations are rarely needed but if there are atypical symptoms then radiological imaging may be helpful. Electromyography of the pelvic floor is used to evaluate muscle tone but is not needed in basic clinical practice.

Diagnosis

It is most important to put patients at ease, showing the ability to listen and communicate. There should be time to allow patients to talk about their symptoms and it is important to acknowledge that they are real. They have often seen other healthcare providers who are unfamiliar with the diagnosis and, as there is nothing to see on examination, this may make them feel as if the symptoms are 'in the head'. Information on lifestyle, personal history, and the effect on their quality of life and relationship is important to evaluate the psychological aspect of the symptoms.

A medical history should establish the first presenting symptom that made them seek medical advice. Patients may be worried that their symptoms indicate malignancy, sexually transmitted infection, or a pathology that no physician can recognize or cure.

Management

There are several treatment options and a multidisciplinary approach is often recommended. It is impossible to define a single therapeutic method that can be used effectively in all women. A patient with vulvodynia has her own history that, if listened to and understood, includes some elements that may guide to the resolution of the problem. Multiple therapeutic approaches have been used in the past (Table 23.1) but some of these are based on minor evidence and have not been subject to rigorous evaluation in double-blind studies. There is a large placebo effect that has been demonstrated in well conducted trials.

In general there are three phases to the management of vulvodynia:

- explanatory phase;
- pharmacological phase;
- psychosexual phase.

The first phase is the consultation, which is most important. The physician should demonstrate a knowledge of the signs, symptoms and management of vulvodynia. An adequate explanation of the condition to the patient often has therapeutic benefits in itself. The explanation should include the types of treatment used including pharmacological and physical therapies, together with the possibility of psychological interventions that may be required.

The pharmacological phase involves topical or systemic treatments as detailed below. Physical therapies such as physiotherapy can be helpful.

Local Topical Pain Modifiers

Local anaesthetics such as 5% lidocaine ointment are most helpful in patients with localized provoked pain resulting in introital dyspareunia. It can be used daily and also before intercourse.

Amitriptyline cream (2%) and 0.025%–0.05% capsaicin cream have also been used but the latter is not well tolerated and causes burning on application.

Systemic Pain Modifiers

Amitriptyline, a tricyclic antidepressant (TCA), can be very useful for its ability to decrease nociceptive transmission in peripheral nerves. Furthermore, it is a potent serotonin-norepinephrine

Table 23.1 Treatments used.

Medical		
Topical	Steroid	
	Antibiotics, antifungals	
	Oestrogens	
Intralesional	Steroid	
	Interferon	
Oral	Tricyclic antidepressants	
	Calcium citrate	
Other	Psychotherapy	
	Biofeedback	
	Acupuncture	
	TENS (transcutaneous electrical nerve stimulation)	
Surgical		
Destructive	Diathermy	
	Cryocoagulation	
	CO_2 laser	
	Argon laser	
Excisional	Vestibulectomy	

reuptake inhibitor in the central nervous system. Nortriptyline is an alternative. Patients are often very sensitive to the side effects of these drugs and therefore a small dose, for example 10 mg, is used and is best taken at night. This can be increased by 10 mg every 3–4 weeks to a maximum of 70–80 mg/day. Larger doses have been used in some studies but the side effects often limit their use. Side effects include drowsiness, dizziness, constipation and occasionally weight gain but these tend to reduce with continuing therapy.

The anticonvulsant gabapentin increases production of the inhibitory neurotransmitter γ-amino butyric acid (GABA) and has been used in the treatment of vulvodynia. The dose recommended is generally 300 mg/day to start and then increasing by 300 mg every week to 1200 mg/day, although some studies increase further to 3000 mg/day. Side effects include drowsiness, fatigue, sleep disturbance and dizziness. There may be an adverse effect on sexual function and reduced orgasm is reported.

Physical Therapy

Chronic vulval pain can lead to changes in the pelvic floor muscles with increased muscle tone. Physiotherapy can be helpful in increasing patients' awareness of this problem and to teach them to fully relax the pelvic floor muscles. It can be particularly helpful for those with significant vaginismus.

Biofeedback is best used by a trained physiotherapist who is experienced in managing these patients.

Other nerve-modulating techniques, such as TENS and nerve blocks, can be used by pain specialists. Some patients find acupuncture helpful.

Psychosexual Therapy

The psychosexual phase relates to treatments based on behavioural, relational and sexual theories. The behavioural approach tries to influence symptoms by teaching modifications of behaviour. These include lifestyle factors but also emotional aspects of pain behaviour. The relational approach explores emotional aspects of relationships and the effect of pain on this. The sexual approach is based on the fact that the vulva is an organ for sexual communication and dysfunction may affect sexual desire. As vulvodynia is a disorder with complex features, the psychologist should adapt to the patient's needs and may need to use a combination approach. Techniques used include cognitive behavioural therapy, couple therapy and mindfulness.

Surgical Treatment

Surgery has been performed in cases where all other treatment has failed. The most common procedure undertaken is a posterior vestibulectomy. Some studies show an improvement in symptoms but the follow up is short and the evidence for long-term benefit is lacking. It has been shown to be less effective than cognitive behavioural therapy. In some cases, surgical intervention can make the pain worse.

Further Reading

Andrews, J. C. (2011) Vulvodynia interventions – systematic review and evidence grading. *Obstetrical and Gynecological Survey* **66**, 299–315.

Haefner, H. K., Collins, M. E., Davis, G. D. *et al.* (2005) The vulvodynia guideline. *Journal of Lower Genital Tract Disease* **9**(1), 40–51.

Mandal, D., Nunns, D., Byrne, M. *et al.* (2010) Guidelines for the management of vulvodynia. *British Journal of Dermatology* **162**, 1180–1185.

Moyal-Barracco, M. and Lynch, P. J.. (2004) 2003 ISSVD terminology and classification of vulvodynia: a historical perspective. *Journal of Reproductive Medicine* **49**, 772–777.

Sadownik, L. A. (2014) Etiology, diagnosis and clinical management of vulvodynia. *International Journal of Women's Health* **6**, 437–449.

Useful Web Sites for Patient Information

British Vulval Pain Society:
www.vulvalpainsociety.org (accessed 14 September 2016)

International Society for Study of Vulvovaginal Disease
www.issvd.org (accessed 14 September 2016)
http://www.issvd.org/issvd-terminology-classification-of-vulvar-diseases/ (accessed 19 September 2016)

National Vulvodynia Association
www.nva.org (accessed 14 September 2016)

24

Psychosexual Aspects of Vulval Disease

The vulva has a complex anatomy and physiology. It belongs to the female reproductive system but the relationship between its structure and its reproductive function cannot be fully understood without integrating the concept that the vulva is also a sexual organ. Its sexual function is not only related to its reproductive function – the vulva also has an important role with regard to intimate communication and sexual arousal. It is an organ linked with an important identity and symbolic meaning. The anthropologists give the vulva – like the penis – a function in social communication.

External sexual organs are connecting organs. A special and intimate connection exists with pleasure and they are at the centre of body identity. The ability to experience one's own sexuality fully is a result of a long learning process, partially conscious and partially unconscious, which continues through the whole lifetime. The fact that the vulva is involved in identity and intimate communication of pleasure has been neglected for a long time. Gynaecologists considered it as the last part of the delivery canal, dermatologists as a remote region of the 'skin planet' and psychologists as a mysterious organ wrapped in emotion. This prevented the creation of specific expertise in this area for a long time. Now there are specialists in sexology and psychosexual disorders who can be very helpful to these patients. The physician should be aware of underlying issues affecting psychosexual health and should refer the patient to an appropriate specialist for expert advice.

Vulval disorders, from the banal to the most serious, therefore have an impact on the psyche and emotional state that can be much more important than with other diseases. This kind of upset has the potential to cause worry and anxiety, which have a significant impact on patients, their partners and their relationships. A mild episode of candidiasis, for instance, will restrict sexual activity. This can lead to an important negative impact on psychosexual quality of life, on relationships and on body image. If recurrent, then at a particular moment of life, or phase of a relationship, it can produce enormous damage and represents a real psychological issue. When the physical problem becomes chronic, then some women start questioning their actions and ask 'Why has all this happened to me?' or 'Where did it come from?' or worse, 'Have I been cheated?' An infection of any other organ would not have such a dramatic impact. Feeling 'infected' or 'guilty' is devastating for sexual health and it is why healthcare workers caring for these patients should pay special attention to these aspects of vulval disease and show sensitivity in dealing with them. It is very common for women to seek consultations with physicians regarding problems related to orgasm and lack of sexual desire and there is a high prevalence of sexual dysfunction in women presenting to vulval clinics. Even more women ask advice for vulval asymmetry or perceived aesthetic defects.

Women have a wide variety of responses when dealing with their own vulval pathology, which can range from apathy, ignoring neoplastic lesions for many years, to great anxiety about mild and benign

A Practical Guide to Vulval Disease: Diagnosis and Management, First Edition. Fiona Lewis, Fabrizio Bogliatto and Marc van Beurden.
© 2017 John Wiley & Sons Ltd. Published 2017 by John Wiley & Sons Ltd.

symptoms. Everyone has some emotional relationship to their genital organs that is related to their own history and personal experience. Each individual has a different capability when facing discomfort and therefore people will react to the same situation in different ways.

There are specific conditions or events that frequently cause psychosexual issues. These include vulval pain, sexual abuse or sexual assault, female genital mutilation and extensive surgical procedures such as vulvectomy for malignancy. However, it is important to remember that the individual response to a problem may mean that psychosexual issues can occur with any vulval problem, however mild it might seem to the physician.

Vaginal and vulval symptoms are frequently present in women with sexual difficulties. The most common are the lack of lubrication due to a reduced sexual interest, lack of desire and lack of fantasies. Another common problem that the vulvologist should be familiar with is vaginismus. This is a neuromuscular defensive reflex that amplifies any discomfort associated with penetration, causing pain.

The definition of female sexual arousal disorder (FSAD) is still debated and it may not exist as a pure entity. It may be an abnormal response that can be influenced by many factors including mood and any difficulties in the relationship with the sexual partner. In the male, physical causes can lead to problems with arousal.

Clinical Psychological Assessment

During the consultation with a patient with vulval symptoms, the physician should take note of nonverbal signs exhibited by the patient, which may indicate anxiety or other psychological issues. These include extreme reserve or difficulty in lying down for examination, the inclination to close the legs, tremor of the hands or voice, excessive sweating or occasionally aggressive behaviour. If detected, then anxiety and other problems can be explored further. It is appropriate to start with a short psychosexual history as long as the patient does not show embarrassment or hostility to it. Questions about sexual satisfaction and desire can give valuable information and this could lead to the discovery of personal unresolved problems such as conflicts with the partner or preconceptions about their problem. If psychosexual issues are discovered, then the patient can be referred for expert advice on further management.

Further Reading

Aerts, L., Enzlin, P., Vergote, I. *et al.* (2012) Sexual, psychological and relational functioning in women after surgical treatment for vulvar malignancy: a literature review. *Journal of Sexual Medicine* **9**, 361–371.

Bergeron, S., Likes, W. M. and Steben, M. (2014) Psychosexual aspects of vulvovaginal pain. *Best Practice and Research: Clinical Obstetrics and Gynecology* **28**, 991–999.

Giraldi, A., Rellini, A. H., Pfaus, J. and Laan, E. Female sexual arousal disorders. *Journal of Sexual Medicine* **10**, 58–73.

Gunzler, C. and Berner, M. M. (2012) Efficacy of psychosocial interventions in men and women with sexual dysfunctions–a systematic review of controlled clinical trials: Part 2 – the efficacy of psychosocial interventions for female sexual dysfunction. *Journal of Sexual Medicine* **9**, 3108–3125.

Gordon, D., Gardella, C., Eschenbach, D. and Mitchell, C. M. (2016) High prevalence of sexual dysfunction in a vulvovaginal specialty clinic. *Journal of Lower Genital Tract Disorders* **20**, 80–84.

25

Benign Lesions

Cysts and other benign lesions related to the vulva are common. A few of the more frequently seen conditions are described here.

Epidermoid Cysts

Epidermoid cysts are very common on the vulva. They are frequently multiple (Figure 25.1), affect the inner and outer labia majora and may extend to the mons pubis. They appear as yellow papules or nodules and may become large (Figure 25.2). No treatment is required but they can be simply excised.

Comedones

If the sebaceous duct related to a hair follicle is blocked by sebaceous material and keratin debris, a comedone results (Figure 25.3). These may open to the surface (blackhead) or closed (whitehead). They become more common on the vulva with increasing age and usually occur on the hair-bearing portion of the labia majora or mons pubis. The contents of open comedones can be expressed but they can refill and recur. Bridged comedones are classic of hidradenitis (see Chapter 14).

Syringomata

These are small, benign, eccrine tumours most commonly seen under the lower eyelids. They are uncommon on the vulva but present as flesh-coloured papules, which are often itchy. The histology is characteristic, showing cystic ductal structres, which have a 'tadpole' appearance. The important differential diagnosis is that of a microcystic adnexal carcinoma.

If asymptomatic, no treatment is needed, but they can be pruritic. Several destructive treatments such as electrodessication and carbon dioxide laser have been used.

A Practical Guide to Vulval Disease: Diagnosis and Management, First Edition. Fiona Lewis, Fabrizio Bogliatto and Marc van Beurden.
© 2017 John Wiley & Sons Ltd. Published 2017 by John Wiley & Sons Ltd.

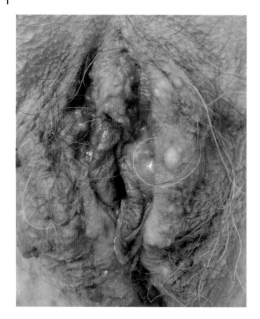

Figure 25.1 Multiple epidermoid cysts.

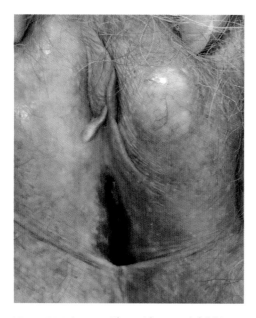

Figure 25.2 Large epidermoid cyst on left labium majus in a patient with lichen planus.

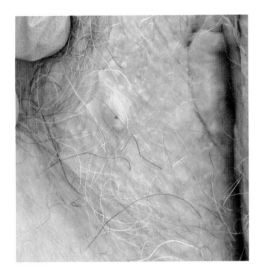

Figure 25.3 Open comedone.

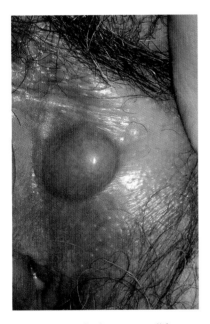

Figure 25.4 Hidradenoma papilliferum.

Hidradenoma Papilliferum

These are benign tumours, probably arising from the ano-genital glands. The most common site is the interlabial sulcus. They are almost exclusively described in Caucasian women. They generally present as mobile, cystic structures (Figure 25.4) but can sometimes ulcerate. Treatment is by simple excision.

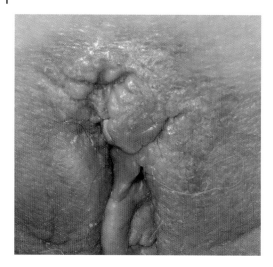

Figure 25.5 Lymphangiectasia in Crohn's disease.

Lymphangioma/Lymphangiectasia

Lymphangiectasia are small, dilated lymphatic channels and can occur as part of a congenital lesion or acquired. They can be related to Crohn's disease (Figure 25.5) or can occur after surgery or infection if there is damage to underlying vessels. The clinical appearance is often described as resembling frog spawn. Recurrent cellulitis can be a complication. Treatment can be complex and patients should be referred to a specialist clinic.

Further Reading

Heller, D. S. (2011) Benign papular lesions of the vulva. *Journal of Lower Genital Tract Disorders* **16**, 1–10.

Huang, Y. H., Chuang, Y. H., Kuo, T. T. *et al.* (2003) Vulvar syringoma: a clinicopathological and immunohistologic study of 18 patients and results of treatment. *Journal of the American Academy of Dermatology* **48**, 735–739.

Index

A Practical Guide to Vulval Disease: Diagnosis and Management, First Edition. Fiona Lewis, Fabrizio Bogliatto
and Marc van Beurden.
© 2017 John Wiley & Sons Ltd. Published 2017 by John Wiley & Sons Ltd.